The South Florida Dental Implant

Patient Guidebook

Teeth in One Day

with Dental Implants

By Matthew J. Holtan, DDS

First Printing: 2020

ISBN 978-1-947744-49-3

Imprint by: Twisted Key Publishing, LLC

Ordering Information:
Special discounts are available on quantity purchases by corporations, associations, educators, and others. For details, contact the publisher at the above listed address.

U.S. trade bookstores and wholesalers: Please contact Twisted Key Publishing, LLC by email twistedkeypublishing@gmail.com.

Dedicated to helping every patient gain clarity and understanding of the life-changing miracles of modern implant dentistry

This guidebook is written for
intended to replace component
related to medical or dental healtl
advised to schedule a consultation
with a licensed physician or dentist.

Table of Contents

Chapter 1 Introduction

- But Then Reality Sets In
- Photos? Not Me!!
- It's Taking a Big Toll on You
- Facing Reality Is What Turns the Corner

Chapter 2 What You Get in This Patient Guidebook

- Just a Few of the Life-Changing Things Modern Dentistry Can Mean for You
- Our Guarantees are Solid
- 22 Types of Patients Who Benefit from Our Method of Implant Dentistry
- A Perfect Example of How Dr. Holtan's Method of Implant Dentistry Can Restore Your Dental Health, Function, and Beauty
- The Proven Solution That Gives a Great Smile and Healthy Teeth for Life
- What if There Was a Type of Dentistry That You Could Experience That...

Chapter 3 How It All Happened

- How a Lucky Break Changed How I Practice Dentistry
- How a Chance Conversation Overheard Led Me to the Secrets of Dental Implant Success...

- They Laughed When I Told Them I Was Studying Dental Implants, but When I Showed Them My Patients, Their Ridicule Turned to Admiration!
- For the Record, You Should Know About Dr. Holtan Too

Chapter 4 Hey, I Just Realized You Might Not Know... What Is A Dental Implant?

- Here's How It Works...
- Types of Dental Implants

  Conventional Dental Implants
  All-on-4 Dental Implants
  The NeoArch Technique-Same Day Teeth
  The Sub-Periosteal Dental Implant
  Mini Dental Implants
  Small Diameter Dental Implants
  Cosmetic Single Front Implant Teeth

Chapter 5 Have You Been Told You Can't Have a Dental Implant?

- Do You Think You'll Suffer with Dentures Forever? You Can't Wear Dentures Another Day? You Can't Smile and Chew Like You Used To?
- Dental Implants Restore Lost Chewing Ability
- Are You Embarrassed to Smile or Open Your Mouth?
- What Happened When They Lost Their Dentures?
- Do You Suffer from These Effects of Missing and Failing Teeth?
- New Research Shows Connection Between Tooth Loss and Slowing Mind

- More Blunt Truth About Missing Teeth

  Missing Teeth Biologically Impair Man
  You Will Need Your Teeth Longer
  Missing Teeth Help Destroy Self-Confidence and
    Change How You Smile
  A Single Missing Tooth Can Cause Damage That
    You Can't Feel or See
  Are You Making This Mistake?
  Diseased Teeth and Gums Threaten Your Health...
    (And Your Family's Health!)

Chapter 6 Do You Love to Eat?

- Why Enjoying the Taste and Experience of Your
  Food Is More Important Than Ever
- Dentures Decrease Function and Chewing Ability
  and Change the Foods You Eat for the Worse
- The Whole-Body Health and Teeth Connection
- Check Your Tongue for Bacteria Right Now!
- Diabetics CAN Save Their Teeth
- Infections in the Mouth Make Other Diseases
  Worse
- Consider Changing Your Oral Hygiene Habits
  TODAY!

Chapter 7 Don't Let Missing Teeth Rob You of the
Pleasures of Living

- Implants Help – A Lot!!
- Missing Teeth Encourage Wrinkling and Premature
  Aging
- WARNING! If You're Considering Plastic
  Surgery, Don't Make This Mistake!

- Partial Dentures Cause Bone Loss, Too!
- Don't Hold onto Diseased Teeth Too Long and Destroy Your Jaw Bones!
- Denture Adhesives Are Not a Good Solution
- An 89% Better Outlook on Life
- Dental Implants Give Predictable Success – Far Better Than Dental Bridges
- Dental Implants Work with a Single or Multiple Missing Teeth
- Almost All People with Missing Teeth Can Benefit from Implants

Chapter 8 Advantages of Dr. Holtan's Method Implant Dentistry

- 30 Advantages of Our Method of Implant Dentistry
- If Dentistry Has Been Difficult for You, You Can Relax!
- Stone Age Dentistry Is a Thing of the Past
- We Are "Armed to the Teeth" with Technology and Techniques for a Better Dental Experience

Chapter 9 Looking Good

- Attractiveness Determines How Other People Perceive and Treat You
- Social Advantages of Looking Good
- An Investment in Yourself
- Implants Make Good Economic Sense
- Prevent Pain, Save Money

Chapter 10 Appointments, Fees, Billing, and Insurance Must Be Easy for You!

- Financing Made Easy
- Why Deal with Insurance Companies Yourself?

Chapter 11 The Horrible Hidden Costs of NOT Doing Treatment

- Enhance Your Career... Make More Money
- A Case of Investing in Yourself
- You're Never Too Old to Have a Healthy Mouth
- It Does Take Time but Less Than You Imagine

Chapter 12 Competence You Can Count On

- Report: What Happens to Patients Who Have Implants
- We Can Be More Than Just Your Implant Dentist

Chapter 13 Is a Smile an Investment That Makes Sense to You?

- Calculate How Much Your Smile Is Worth

Chapter 14 People Always Look at Your Teeth... What Do They See?

- Attractiveness Determines How Others Perceive and Treat You in All Situations

Chapter 15 Three More Ways a Great Smile Can Influence Your Day

- Social Advantages of Looking Good and Having a Great Smile

- Attractive School Children Get into Less Trouble and Are Seen as Being Smarter
- Good-Looking Political Candidates Are More Likely to Win Elections

Chapter 16 Four More Ways a Great Smile Influences Your Life

- Being Attractive Makes Getting Jobs Easier
- Attractiveness Influences the Law and Justice System
- You Can Make More Money if You Have a Great Smile
- Men and Women Agree That Attractive Teeth Are Better

Chapter 17 Not Having a Good-Looking Smile Used to Be Optional – Not Anymore

- You Can Even Help Someone You Care About – Here's How

Chapter 18 Shocking News – All Dentists Don't Use the Latest Techniques

- Not All Dentists Are the Same!
- Your Childhood Dentist Is an Example
- Not All Dentists Provide Celebrity Smiles
- Dentists May Specialize in Traumatic, Serious Cases
- Consider Your State of Oral Health Right Now

Chapter 19 Six Considerations to Make When Choosing a Dentist

- You Need a Dentist Who Is Savvy About Dental Advancements
- You Need a Dentist Who Can Make Complex Dentistry Simple to Understand

Chapter 20 Make Sure the Initial Visit Is Free

- You Shouldn't Have to Pay for the First Visit
- Your First Visit Is Similar to a Date in Some Ways
- Then You Have to Enforce Your Beliefs
- If There's No Evidence of These Two Things at the First Visit, Move on to Another Practice
- Get a Guarantee from Your Dentist
- What You Really Want at Any Dental Office
- No Scolding and No Embarrassment – Guaranteed
- "Can't Go Wrong" First Complete Dental Physical Examination – Guaranteed or It's Free

Chapter 21 Make Sure Your Dentist Has a Proven Track Record

- Three Types of People & Three Types of Dentists
- The Type #2 Dentist (The Average Dentist) – Not for Those with Major Problems
- The Bottom Line Is Your Mouth Is Different
- The Type #3 Dentist – The Expert Level Dentist

Chapter 22 Work with as Few Dentists as Possible

- There Are Highly Qualified Type #3 Expert Dentists

- Your Biggest Non-Recoverable Asset Is Always Your Time
- Full-Service Dentistry Is Available
- Why Not Have One All-Encompassing Dentist?

Chapter 23 Find a Dentist Who Makes Office Procedures Easy

- Your New Dentist's Business Office Should be Administratively Painless
- We Often Find That Patients Don't Understand Their Dental Insurance Policies
- We Guarantee to Maximize Your Insurance

Chapter 24 Make Sure Your Dentist Talks About Your Teeth for the Rest of Your Life

- How to Find a Dentist Who Thinks About Your Teeth from a Long-Term Perspective
- What Should Happen at Your First Visit?
- A Dental Examination Is an Important Part of the Appointment
- You Have a Right to Know the Best Options
- Every Dentist, Including Us, Is Not Right for Everyone

Chapter 25 Find a Dentist Within a Reasonable Travel Distance

- Beware of "Vacation" Dentistry
- The Bottom Line on Choosing a Dentist

Chapter 26 Dental Implants – An Investment in Yourself That You Deserve

- Most People Have No Idea of Just How Important Their Teeth Are!

*Think about the difference between a mountain climber who has mastered the skill of summiting the world's tallest mountain peaks and a novice. The difference in skill, ability, and thought process is immense! Solving complex dental needs are as technical or <u>even more so</u> than any mountain climbing expedition. Wouldn't you prefer that your dental care come from those with a level of mastery who can focus their talents on <u>**you**</u> just as much as a skilled master climber focuses on summiting the world's most formidable peaks?*

Dr. Holtan is such a master and has an amazing dedication to dentistry. His commitment to providing the best for his patients is exemplified by the amazing smiles he creates and the comfort he brings to those needing major dental treatment. From Dr. Holtan, you can expect excellent results that help you chew comfortably and enjoy what modern dentistry can do. All you need to do is to allow him to focus his world-class expert skills for your personal benefit.

— Dr. James R. McAnally, Clinician and Top Advisor to the Profession

Chapter 1
Introduction

Dazzle Your Smile...Supercharge Your Sex Appeal....Feel Whole Again...Regain Lost Function...Get Noticed by That Special Someone...Save Your Health and Live Longer...Get Back a Youthful Vibrancy...Look and Feel 10-20 Years Younger...

These requests we hear in our office all the time are surprisingly easy to accomplish when one thing is changed – the teeth. How can that be, you might ask?

Let's take the case of someone who has had a missing tooth for a while. If this is you, you can relate. At first, you're super conscious about that missing tooth. You get comments about it and it's not pleasant.

You also can't help noticing that there are others who don't kid you about missing a tooth but are staring at the area of your mouth where

1

the tooth was. These are the "nice" people who don't want you to feel embarrassed – but you still do feel embarrassed.

You begin to adapt. When you smile, you don't show the bottom or upper teeth, whichever part of your mouth that has the missing tooth. You start to avoid social situations both at work and even with family. You dread being on the scene of any major event. What if a news crew shows up and they happen to select you as that wise innocent bystander? Needless to say, your self-esteem would be at stake and put on display. Who wants to take those kinds of chances?!?

But Then Reality Sets In

Over time, you realize you're almost becoming a shut-in. And then if this period of time goes on for far too long, you notice that you're really missing out on a lot of life as a result. If you're single, you aren't meeting people or dating, and life is a lot less passionate without someone special in your life; even if it's simply a friend to enjoy time and activities with.

If you're married, you notice that your spouse isn't kissing you as much anymore, too. You rationalize it in your mind from the one comment she (or he) made that your mouth feels strange without the tooth, but whatever reason, it's not pleasant.

Photos? Not Me!!

The worst-case scenario is when you attend get-togethers and people bring out their cell phones to take photos. It's not as bad because you learned "how to smile" less to hide the empty space after about a month. These days everyone has not only cameras but also video cameras in their phones and they love to use them.

What if your smile shows the missing tooth? Then this whole bad situation will be passed on in photos or video footage for who knows how long! Your whole family will say, "Oh yeah, the one without the tooth!" or something else not so nice. Once the cameras are pulled out of pockets and purses, that's when many people who are missing teeth will run and hide, as if they were a little dog who did something bad and the master comes home.... Heaven forbid if the photo or video gets "shared" on Facebook!

It's Taking a Big Toll on You

You may not realize it but this whole issue about not having a tooth – or several teeth

– or any teeth really does take a toll on you. If left to continue, the loss of several teeth will even start to change the shape of the face, making you look much older than your actual years.

The teeth play a big role in your attractiveness – and as you know, our society judges people by how they look much of the time! We'll explore and expand on the role our teeth and smiles make in our lives that most people, including members of the dental profession, are unaware of in this patient guidebook.

And then there are the creeping diet changes you make. Many people who lost a few teeth can't chew as well as they used to, so they forgo the healthy salads and their favorite cuts of meat – replacing them with softer foods and more processed foods. Before long, they find new health symptoms that are the result of vitamin and mineral deficiencies. Most never connect the dots between the gradual change in diet related to the teeth *and* the health symptoms.

The change to softer, more processed foods also means a switch to foods higher in salt and sugar. Now we're headed down the path of developing high blood pressure and diabetes, two killer diseases that can dramatically shorten lifespans. Later in this guidebook, we'll explain some of the recent studies of what happens to the health of people who lose a tooth or teeth. Your schoolteacher in health class probably didn't tell you that every tooth is ultimately connected to the health of our organs since this information is so new. We'll cover the most important things to know related to the mouth-body-health connection.

Facing Reality Is What Turns the Corner

There comes a time when you have to admit that you can't win this battle. You simply have to replace the missing tooth or teeth so you can get on with your life.

Here's the missing piece of information you didn't know before – modern implant dentistry has made this process SO EASY that you will kick yourself when you find out about it, and say, "Why didn't I do it before? Why did I put myself through all this grief when I didn't have to suffer needlessly or as much as I did?!?"

You're not living in the dentistry days of the 1970s, 1990s, or even early 2000s anymore. Those were the days long before tooth whitening and cosmetic dentistry; when only a

5

rare few of those past the age of 45 had pearly whites. Those were the days of dentures that sat out in a cup next to the person's bedside and frightened all the grandchildren.

The newest and most important technologies that matter the most to you or any patient missing teeth started arriving around 2003 – in particular technologies that create much more speed (so you are in and out of the office in as little time as possible) and accuracy (ensuring better results than at any time in the past).

Everywhere you look technology has made our lives both better but also more confusing. Few in our profession have adopted the technologies that matter the most to you and even fewer realize it's their professional responsibility to make decision making understandable and easy for you the patient when it comes to these advancements.

Part of our role as skilled professionals and something we take great pride in is the ability to make anything that is confusing about your dental choices simple to understand. We realize that as a direct result of making this understandable that more patients will decide to do good things for themselves.

Here are just a few examples of what's happened in less than 10 years:

- You can get a new crown over your lunch break.

- You can also get a dental implant, which is a replacement tooth, in about the same amount of time.

- With a little more time than a lunch break, you can have an entire mouth of new teeth fully supported by "rock-solid" dental implants or a new smile.

- You can have dingy, nicotine-stained, or coffee-stained teeth in the morning and have a smile so white in the afternoon that it scares the cat when the sun sets.

Yes, at times, a bit of humor is necessary to lighten up what is generally a sad topic – stories of patients not getting the best that dentistry can offer due to lapses in professional responsibility for creating understanding.

Your ancestors (not to mention kings, queens, and royalty of all kind) would be truly jealous of the opportunities that are before you and other common, everyday people in the field of dentistry right now – and all you have to do is take advantage of them. We're here to help make the choices understandable.

We wrote this advanced patient guidebook for a few different reasons. These include the following:

✓ Over the years, we have found that there's a lot of confusion about what's possible with dental implants and the options. Thus, this guide was written to reduce confusion on what's possible. We know that confusion means fewer patients making good decisions and spending unnecessary years delaying getting help.

✓ We also realize that for a number of patients who find this guide, they'll have their dentistry done in whatever part of the world they live in as a direct consequence of their better understanding. While we frequently help coordinate schedules for patients traveling long distances inside North America to see us, not everyone can make that journey. Rest assured, we still gain immense professional satisfaction knowing that these unseen patients will receive help from our efforts too. If you are one of these patients, we'd love to hear from you!

✓ Unfortunately, patients are still being told they can't have dental implants by greatly misinformed members of the profession. This "you can't have implants" is simply no longer true, no matter what your situation, thanks to the advancements in dentistry, and especially our unique approach.

✓ There's also a lot of misinformation about what's possible in one day. And then a lot of the time, the information on what these possibilities are is far too technical for the public to understand! That's why we made this book very conversational. If you can't understand, then you will stay confused – and won't do anything about serious dental problems when you could have solid teeth on the very same day, enjoying life more fully again, and with the least amount of time spent needlessly at the dentist. Life's too short to be confused and unable to make a decision!

We'll discuss the pros and cons of current treatments, how dental implants have changed other patients' lives. You'll find out about this brand new way we're approaching dental implants where you can come into the office in the morning and leave with teeth on your dental implants in the afternoon.

If you or a loved one has problem teeth or missing teeth, we want you to know about your options so you can make better choices.

Read on and find out more because your life is about to change into something you have always dreamed of. And tonight when you lay your head to rest on your pillow, you may notice a big difference – instead of sighing about another day gone by, you may be filled with a new sense of hope, one that activates all your dreams of the past. It's a good place to be.

And of course, all those other benefits mentioned in the beginning can soon be converted from negative to positive literally overnight...

Chapter 2
What You Get in This Patient Guidebook

Avoid Embarrassment...Energize Your Relationships...Eat the Foods You Want...Chew Comfortably and Confidently...Rekindle Romance...Live a Longer Life...Preserve Your Health...Get Teeth That Look Good and Feel Good for A Lifetime...

Just a Few of the Life-Changing Things

Modern Dentistry Can Mean for You

This patient guidebook will detail the exciting new advancements in the technologically advanced field of implant dentistry. It reveals the amazing secrets of dental implants, the modern miracle that is bringing renewed smiles to the faces of patients from all over the world.

You'll also find out how other people perceive your smile, why a great smile is important for every aspect of your life, and how to choose a dentist who is truly on your side and can fix your smile the right way.

In this guidebook we will present our case that **you can have the smile you've always wanted,** "ridding yourself of dental handicaps" and getting teeth that look good, feel good, and chew comfortably while **wiping out a serious unknown threat to how long you live and the quality of your life** – and all with one decision – fully supported by a proven system of dental therapy developed over years of advanced training and real world experience: The Dr. Holtan Method of Implant Dentistry.

We urge you to give this your serious and thorough consideration. We honestly believe it could very well be the information you need to know that *could mean all the difference in your life.* If this sounds like outrageous hype, we understand – yet we assure you it is true, and we can prove it.

Our Guarantees Are Solid

We can't guarantee dental implants will change your life. But we can guarantee **that it has changed many of our patients' lives dramatically** for the better.

We can guarantee you need to know the full implication of the detrimental (and often <u>devastating</u>) effects that dental handicaps and diseases, missing teeth, unattractive smiles, and poorly functioning chewing mechanisms have on the quality of your life. It may sound exaggerated, but we assure you it's true.

22 Types of Dental Patients Who Benefit from Dr. Holtan's Method of Implant Dentistry

1) Anyone who wants to preserve their remaining teeth while replacing the missing ones.

2) Denture wearers frustrated and tired of the problems of full dentures and partial dentures...sick of the goo...the pain...the **embarrassment of teeth that can literally fall out in their dinner plate.**

3) Those with bone loss that is causing <u>loss of support for the face</u> or causing an ***ugly, disfiguring appearance*** to the face.

4) Those who have missing teeth or those about to lose teeth due to decay or fracture.

5) Accident victims who want to regain function and appearance.

6) Those who want leading edge technology and techniques.

7) Those who have just "had it" with their deteriorating teeth.

8) If you find you are stuck in a never-ending cycle of crowns, root canals, extractions, and bridges.

9) Those whose teeth are otherwise perfect – except for just one or two missing teeth.

10) Those committed **to a high level of dental health**.

11) Those with a mouthful of problems that just seem to get worse and worse.

12) Those with dentures that "float around," displacing at the worst possible times (also known as *Murphy's Law of Denture Movement –it occurs when the greatest chance of embarrassment is at hand!*).

13) Those considering missing tooth replacement of any kind.

14) **Those that have significant gum disease**.

15) Those disappointed with earlier attempts to fix their teeth.

16) Those considering major dental work.

17) Those with replacement bridges they really don't like having.

18) Those <u>who don't want removable teeth at all</u>.

19) Those who deserve the best dentistry has to offer for the problems of missing teeth.

20) Those who want to recapture their youthful appearance.

21) Those who don't want to experiment with removable teeth. Those who want common sense answers to their functional and appearance related problems.

Were you on the list? Are you a candidate to benefit from the new advancements in dental health?

A Perfect Example of How Dr. Holtan's Method of Implant Dentistry Can Restore Your Dental Health, Function, and Beauty

*I found Dr. Holtan by doing research online. I did so, looking for him through a professional association for implant dentistry. I did that because I had worked in the past for a professional dentist who was a specialist in another community and knew I needed to look at **credentials**.*

When I came to this office, I was overwhelmed by the courtesy, compassion and the professionalism. I just felt at home. I came because I needed some implants and Dr. Molzan (Dr. Holtan's previous partner) was more than wonderful in doing my upper right teeth. I also needed to have some additional work done but I needed to wait a bit. I had been a patient of Dr. Molzan's for 10 years, so when I met Dr. Holtan, who is a younger gentleman, I was delighted. He has the same kind of qualities that Dr. Molzan has.

He did a full restoration of the rest of my mouth on the very front where I had face planted while I was running and damaged my whole lower jaw. I had a lot of wear on my teeth, as well as the damage from my running injury so when I looked in the mirror, I looked kind of worn out, and older.

Plus, I was biting the inside of my lips, which is not a good thing to do, you can create all sorts of problems health wise by doing that. When I had the procedures done, I was so comfortable and was so relaxed that I didn't need sedation, and I actually fell asleep in the chair. It was delightful. Now when I go to the gym, or out with my friends, even my Facebook friends I get nothing but compliments. I smile more, not to mention I can chew better.

My husband had dental phobia but because of my experiences, he's started coming here as a patient and he loves it, he likes coming to the dentist!!! In fact, if I had another mouth, I would do it all over again.

– Trudy

The Proven Solution That Gives a Great Smile and

Healthy Teeth for Life

There are a lot of dental problems that people suffer from needlessly. Let's talk about them, to lay the groundwork for the advancements to solve the relentless problems of missing teeth. Dental implants are:

- A <u>solution</u> to virtually everything that people say they dislike about their teeth and their dental experiences.

- A proven solution <u>to virtually every anxiety that threatens to prevent you from receiving dental care as frequently as you should</u>.

- A solution that provides you with the chance to **reclaim your dental health, to recover from neglect, injury, or bad luck of your draw in the gene pool**.

17

However, this improvement – your dental health – is only one advantage of what we propose to you here.

What if

There Was a Type of Dentistry That You Could Experience That...

✓ Would *virtually guarantee* you a better dental experience

✓ Gives you a vibrant youthful smile you can be proud of

✓ Allows you to have gentle, comfortable dental care

✓ Affords you the opportunity to chew comfortably ***without worry of embarrassing moments***

✓ Frees you from the dental diseases that <u>threaten your longevity</u> and <u>the longevity of your loved ones</u> (**this is astonishing data you must know**)

✓ Is designed especially for your needs and to complete treatment in as few visits as possible

✓ Allows you to sleep well at night, secure in the knowledge you have received state-of-the-art dentistry based on the latest scientifically proven research

✓ Gives **you teeth that feel good and look good and were designed to stay that way**

If all of that actually existed – how interested in it would you be?

How willing would you be to set aside past experiences and ingrained beliefs and habits to seriously consider a new and better way to reclaim or maintain your dental health?

How much is that worth to you?

Before you attempt to come up with or place any mental or monetary value on this, it's vitally important for you to know its true value to your everyday health, well-being, and happiness, all of which we will review in this guidebook.

I found Dr. Holtan thru the newspaper ad regarding dentures. I was more surprised and heartened that he had a straightforward approach, he delivered everything he promised and more. I love my teeth.

I got married since getting my teeth, I don't know if the new teeth helped me get married or not, but if you want the very best, come see Dr. Holtan.

– Dave

Chapter 3
How It All Happened

I want to tell you my story... how I came to know the secrets of dental implant dentistry and my personal struggle to find the truth.

–Dr. Matthew Holtan

How a Lucky Break Changed How I Practice Dentistry

– As told by Dr. Holtan

I'll never forget that day. I was halfway through dental school at Marquette university. All of us (students) were ushered into a lecture hall and given "the talk." A series of our professors flashed slides of dental implants for over an hour showing why, even though the earliest reports coming in from the profession were positive and that dental implants worked, we shouldn't do or consider dental implants in our practices! We were told they were too confusing and too complex to be a routine treatment for all but a small handful of patients.

It struck me as quite strange <u>to wait</u> until this point in our dental careers to discuss a new technology in such a fashion especially considering the immense hope this new development would mean for those with missing teeth The more I revisit this day in my mind, the more shocked I am by the events that transpired!

I immediately recognized this was a subject that I <u>had to know more about</u>. I had to find out the truth about dental implants.

*I recognized that dental implants, <u>if they worked</u>, solved problem after problem after problem. **Missing teeth were and <u>still are</u> a HUGE problem for millions** of patients!*

I began searching. The information written about them at this point in the profession was scant; a small crowd of dentists on the leading edge of the science were reporting that they were known to work and work quite well under the right circumstances. Why had so little education about this developing miracle that held such promise for solving so many of the problems in ways that were better than what we were being taught in dental school?!? I asked doctors whom I knew at other schools and found that everyone was being told the same thing.

I finished my requirements in dental school much sooner than expected and knew I had to find out more about implants. Since my university did not have a post-graduate program for surgical specialists, the full-time faculty specialists did most of the advanced operations in the afternoons. I soon figured out that they would love to teach me any advanced concept I was interested in.

While my classmates took afternoons off to go skiing or to play sports outside (depending on which Wisconsin season we were in), I was assisting experienced clinicians perform complex implant procedures and becoming very familiar with their benefits!

After I graduated, I began searching and found other dentists who had formed into small, special groups to study and help each other with the proper use of implants. That's when I met many of those who would go on to write the textbooks on the subject and to lay the groundwork for what every dentist would eventually be taught.

I was even so fascinated by implant dentistry that I joined a very special organization, the American Academy of Implant Dentistry, which is solely dedicated to spreading the message about implants to the profession and to patients. Ultimately, I would be recognized with the highest educational honors awarded related to implants; awards that less than 0.10% of the profession now hold.

How a Chance Conversation Overheard Led Me to the Secrets of Dental Implant Success...

Serendipity, or random fortuitous events, has struck over and over again. During my senior year of dental school, I traveled to Naples, Florida to visit my grandparents. My grandma handed me a flyer in the local newspaper that advertised advanced implant dentistry by a local doctor. Being an inquisitive, soon-to-be doctor, I called the number in the ad and asked if the doctor would allow me to come and observe while on vacation. The receptionist informed me that would be just fine and two days later there I was, in the Naples, Florida office of Dr. Arthur Molzan.

*The visit with Dr. Molzan was an answer to a prayer. We spent the entire day doing surgery and talking about treatments. He showed me dozens of cases with long-term follow-ups. I almost couldn't believe what I was seeing – **case after case of <u>successful</u> implant treatment lasting years and years**. I felt*

24

electrified... Here was someone who knew! Maybe I could learn from him?

Ultimately, I accepted a position with Dr. Molzan after graduating from dental school, and the rest is history.

Dr. Matthew Holtan graduated from Marquette University with a Bachelor of Science in Biological Sciences and later graduated again with his degree in Dentistry. Dr. Holtan received the American Academy of Implant Dentistry's Student Achievement award and developed an early interest in dental implant therapy. He is a graduate of the AAID Maxicourse in Implant Dentistry and received his training in parenteral conscious sedation from the University of Alabama, Birmingham.

Dr. Holtan is a Fellow of the American Academy of Implant Dentistry and a Diplomate in the American Board of Oral Implantology, which signifies Board Certification in Implant Dentistry. Dr. Holtan has focused his time and energy in helping patients transition from dentures or a terminal dentition into a fixed/permanent replacement solution. In most cases, this is done using a SameDay Approach. He has spoken professionally and has traveled the world seeking the most advanced treatment solutions for his patients.

They Laughed When I Told Them I Was Studying Dental Implants, but When I Showed Them My Patients, Their Ridicule Turned to Admiration!

Dr. Holtan's Personal Story continues…

When my colleagues heard about all my studies on dental implants, they looked at me and shook their heads disapprovingly. I had to suffer "the looks," the whispered comments behind my back, and the general "you're wasting your time and your money." I even got, "How could you do that to your patients?!"

They had been "brainwashed" in dental school. I braved out the looks, the comments, doubts, and negativity of my peers. I knew this was the right thing to do. My convincing arguments, however, fell on deaf ears.

So, I trained...and trained some more. I burned the midnight oil studying my texts and notes. I started doing cases.

*I rejoiced in my successes, and so did my grateful patients who desperately needed what I had to offer: **implant dentistry the right way**.*

My original cases I did are still working, helping my patients smile easily and chew comfortably.

I have been studying what works and what doesn't work ever since. I perform implant dentistry in all its aspects, surgical placement and replacement of missing teeth on a daily basis. The latest developments discussed in this guidebook like the "All-on-4" and "The Sclar Technique" all evolved from the same roots that I've been proud to have been involved in from the very beginning.

I am a bit unusual in that respect.

It is hard to find a practitioner properly schooled and experienced at this level and with this history in <u>both placement and restoration of dental implants</u>. I am proud and pleased to be one of those who lived through the years of skepticism to see the power dental implants have to help people live more fulfilled lives...

*For patients, it means having to **go to only one place to get the work done** instead of being shuffled back and forth between someone who places dental implants and someone else to put on the teeth. It also means that when a technology can predictably allow for speeding up the process of treatment, it will be used for your benefit.*

My colleagues now look at my work with awe and admiration. It took years to happen but eventually those questions of "Why waste time on this new unproven fad?" have been replaced by things like "Wow.... You can do that? That's great" and "What a wonderful service for patients!"

I smile now, knowing I did the right thing. Now – and with each passing year – the profession accepts dental implants as The Answer to Missing Teeth.

For the Record, You Should Know About Dr. Holtan

When Dr. Matthew Holtan graduated from the Marquette University School of Dentistry, he knew he was in the exact profession where he could do the most good in life. He also knew that he wanted to help those patients who needed the best that modern dentistry could do.

While dentistry and dentist's thoughts on dental implants have shifted dramatically over the past 20 years, the reality is that most dental schools, even in 2020, still lag behind the science of the best uses of this amazing technology.

In Dr. Holtan's words,

*During my residency at **Marquette University School of Dentistry**, I was told that* *implants worked very well with over 90% success rates but that they still really weren't for everyone. Looking back this is baffling considering where the science stands, as you will find in this guidebook.*

Fortunately, after my residency, I came into contact with Dr. Molzan, whom I believe is one of the foremost implant dentists based on his history and experience. I immediately realized that I needed to study under him to learn everything I could about this modern miracle.

Dr. Molzan has been doing implants for 30 years with much success! He became my mentor and partner in practice with a goal to help carry forward everything he had learned and help develop in this exciting area.

Since then I've continued learning, have attended over 400 hours of expert level continuing education hours, applied to the American Academy of Implant Dentistry, and have now been named an Associate Fellow of the organization. Fortunately, this organization is at the forefront of the science and information about implants. Each of my patients can count on our combined efforts to give them the best that science and experience can offer to solve their individual problems regardless of how serious they might be.

From his story, you can see that when you decide to get your missing teeth replaced at the dental office of Dr. Holtan, you will benefit from many, many hours of knowledge, wisdom, and experience and are literally in some of the most expert of hands for your dental care in Southwest Florida.

In this life, each thing prepares us for the next. I desperately needed implants. My upper bridge had broken. I endured 3 years with 2 different clumsy partial dentures. I was miserable. I didn't enjoy smiling or eating. It was a nightmare caused by an auto accident 35 years before.

Implants can be too much, an overwhelming, grueling and technical decision. I believe Dr. Matthew Holtan to be the answer in Southwest Florida. He is kind, caring and fun. He listened to me and heard my pain. Putting a lot of compassion into his professional, creative and gifted way, he got through to me

I had 3 implants placed with 6 crowns to correct my dental problem. Also, his hygienist did a cleaning which was more thorough than I've ever had before. It was wonderful! I heartily recommend Dr. Holtan and his staff.

– Deborah B., Naples, FL

Chapter 4
Hey, I Just Realized You Might Not Know...What Is A Dental Implant?

A dental implant is a biologically compatible, man-made substitute to replace missing tooth roots; it is usually made of a space-age alloy mostly of titanium. Implants come in various shapes and sizes to fit the situation. Most are cylinder shaped when placed into bone and allowed to heal undisturbed while bone heals around them, locking them in like an anchor. After a few months, the implants are used as a foundation for replacing the missing teeth. This describes the way the majority of professionals still operate when it comes to dental implant therapies.

If months seems like a long time to you, rest assured we feel the same way and there is some great news in this respect to time. Thanks to new science in use at Dr. Holtan's, we can speed this process up so that

transitional teeth are attached to the implants the same day instead of waiting months! We'll get into this breakthrough – including a discussion about The Sclar "One Day" Technique and other advancements – later in the guidebook.

Dental implants <u>restore</u> lost chewing ability, <u>improve appearance</u>, <u>end embarrassment</u>, and <u>give real self-confidence</u> to patients who need them. They are a real breakthrough!

Here's How It Works...

The steps of the implant procedure itself are quite simple:

1) If there is a damaged tooth, it is painlessly removed.

2) The actual "implant," a small titanium post, is implanted into your actual jawbone.

   The thickness and type of bone at the implant's location determine which style should be used. Local anesthesia and Dr. Holtan's gentle techniques make this a **VERY** comfortable process.

3) Your body immediately begins to "bond" the titanium into place with your bone or tissue. This is a very thorough process and may take

from one to six months. Again, this is describing "classic" dental implant therapy and we will go into the new methods in use at Dr. Holtan's that greatly speed up treatment a bit later.

No matter what version of therapy you choose, your body does not reject these new materials but ties them in with great strength as if they were a natural part of your own body. During the process, you always have some type of teeth over the implants.

In the newest methods used at Dr. Holtan's, patients are able to leave the office on the same day as surgery with teeth solidly in place on the implants, which most patients find appealing.

4) Once the titanium implant is tightly in place, a tooth can be directly attached to the titanium implant and you can begin functioning with the new teeth immediately!

5) You have a new tooth. You are the only one who knows it's man- made – and implants are so comfortable you'll soon forget which one it is.

Your body thinks it's your own – so will you!

Dental implants are the most stable and economically far-sighted solution to the very real problem of missing teeth. This procedure is one which we have done repeatedly for satisfied patients over many years. Our friendly staff also has in-depth training and great experience in this area and will be happy to answer any questions that you may have.

Read on about the other types of dental implants here and you'll be able to converse with your dentist about them. After a discussion on what your needs and desires are with treatment, a competent Expert level Type #3 dentist will help guide you through choices that will work for your situation. Later in the guidebook you'll find a thorough discussion on how to determine the level of expertise of any dentist you may be considering entering into a discussion with about your situation.

Types of Dental Implants

There are several types of dental implants, and the more you know about them, the more you can discuss them with your dentist with whom you may be contemplating treatment. The five different types of dental implants are: 1) Conventional implants, 2) All-on-Four dental implants, 3) The NeoArch

Technique-Same Day Teeth), 4) Sub-Periosteal implants, and 5) Mini implants.

Conventional Dental Implants

Conventional dental implants work, and have worked for years, but the problem is that many people don't want to wait to get them – or can't get them for various reasons! As mentioned previously, with the "classic" or conventional method of treatment there is a period of time (2-6 months) when nothing is attached to the implants.

Your particular situation will dictate which implants will work best in which scenarios. Typically, if a patient is only replacing a few back (molar) teeth, we must give the body a short period of time to heal the titanium implants BEFORE delivering the permanent teeth.

All-on-4 Dental Implants

The total cost of a dental implant or dental implants is more than simply the bottom-line cost of what you invest in treatment out of your own pocket. There's the cost of healing time, the cost of pain and embarrassment of not having teeth, cost of actual pain inflicted by practices not concerned with patient comfort during the procedure, cost of care of any products for the teeth, and the personal and emotional well-being cost. There's also the nutritional cost that must be calculated in the big picture, as missing teeth clearly can be a cause of nutritional deficiencies, creating or contributing to other cascading health issues.

One of the types of dental implants that can save money and time is the All-on-4 procedure. This procedure is one of the more minimally invasive solutions with a fixed full arch of teeth. This procedure may be perfect for those who:

• have no teeth

• have failing teeth (teeth that are broken down and in need of constant repair)

• are wearing dentures

• need full upper and/or lower restorations

Traditional dental implants used to replace an entire jaw (top or bottom) require 6 to 8 implants, or more depending on the current status of the teeth, whereas the All-on-4 procedure uses only 4 special type of implants designed for this procedure. It offers a full set of teeth per arch, and each arch of teeth is supported by these 4 highly specialized implants.

Here's the most important part of the process: you can usually get the procedure completed in one dental visit. This means you walk out of our dental office with real teeth, ready for strong, biting action. The bite strength improves 70+% with the All-on-4 procedure because of the angle of the implants. Following the one-day procedure, a second set of permanent teeth is eventually attached after there has been complete healing, about 6 to 8 months after surgery. During this time, most find the teeth they left with on the day of surgery feeling so solid they are surprised that there is a next step.

There are other benefits you should know about:

- These implants may be cleaned like your regular teeth.

- They don't cause pain by compressing your gums since nothing is moving.

- They don't need any type of dental adhesives.

- They assist in preventing bone deterioration of the jaw, unlike dentures. The implants are placed at an angle so there is greater contact with bone.

- It provides more support for facial tissues that can improve appearance.

- These are very stable implants.

- You don't need bone grafting or other extensive surgical procedures that add risk and discomfort for the All-on-4 procedure.

This procedure has already been proven to be highly successful by dental researchers. Specifically, the rate of success is 98% for long-term, 5 to 10 years of usage.

In one long-term study, 95% of 250 patients were satisfied with their new teeth, and 74% of them were extremely satisfied. In contrast, less than 5% of denture wearers are satisfied with their teeth. That's up to a 1900% change in satisfaction level thanks to this exciting development!

The NeoArch Technique-Same Day Teeth

This revolutionary advancement beyond the All-on-4 method came into being in 2013 and is now in use by roughly 70 dentists worldwide, including Dr. Holtan. It allows for far more flexibility, allowing for additional implants beyond four, if and when needed, for a specific patient's situation. It also gets you back to living life at its fullest in the shortest amount of time.

In the NeoArch Technique, a special type of x-ray scan allows us to create a 3-D image of what is happening in your mouth and when possible keeps the gums from needing to be cut open. Anywhere from a few days to a few weeks later, dependent on how fast the patient needs or desires to return after the 3-D scan is performed, the new teeth will be waiting to be placed – again when possible without a gum flap surgery. This procedure can be less invasive than any other previous way of performing dental implants. Less invasive means less discomfort. In fact, *with a specific regimen of treatment and medications*, patients report virtually no pain.

There is often a waiting list to get into the training for this advancement in implant therapy as only so many dentists can be capably trained in the technique each year. Because of the fact that few dentists can be trained each year, for most readers of this guidebook, it is unlikely they will find a local dentist performing the NeoArchTechnique. For those who desire this advancement and who will need to travel, our team can and will help make arrangements so that you too can benefit.

No matter what type of dental implant you ultimately get, most patients will want one of these newer techniques that dramatically shorten the amount of time in treatment and shorten the number of visits. Procedures that took months to complete can now be condensed into a matter of hours or days thanks to advanced x-ray scans, 3-D modeling, and computer-aided design, especially when these technologies are in the right expert's hands. We are proud to be pioneering dentists in South Florida, bringing these advancements to the general public and for the benefit of our patients.

But there is one major problem with these new techniques. It has to do with patients not deciding to move forward with this type of care. You see, the longer you wait, the greater your chances of not being eligible for the newer techniques at the fastest treatment speeds possible.

Beyond this major problem, there is also another reason not to procrastinate with getting the help you need. Due to the great public demand from patients needing the All-on-4 and NeoArch Technique coupled with our current obligations to present patients, there is simply not enough time in a given year to treat all of those desiring these newest methods. Thus, the sooner you personally have a consultation the better.

You also should really see how life-changing dental implant technology really is. There are always new patient stories and photos of patients who felt that they "couldn't be fixed" at www.NoMoreDentures.net.

For those who felt that life was hopeless dentally, they are so glad they were wrong – and they are living life to the fullest every minute. Please take a few minutes to visit the website and have a look at these patients and their stories. Imagine the difference in how people perceive them now – all from Dr. Holtan's Method of Implant Dentistry. They made up for the ravages of time or unfortunate accidents and so can you!

It is very likely you also know others who desperately need either the All-on-4 or The Sclar "One Day" Technique – and they need to know there is still hope for them. Please share this info with them and share the web address so they can also see what is possible. Often if we don't see what's possible, we can't imagine how things could be different!

And by the way, our office has literally moved mountains and found new financial options so you can get this type of care. We pride ourselves at coming up with financial solutions for almost every patient who wants the procedure done correctly and is a good candidate for one of these newer implant advancements.

The Sub-Periosteal Dental Implant

The sub-periosteal dental implant is one made out of metal (titanium or chrome, cobalt, and molybdenum). It is attached underneath your gums and rests above or on the jawbone itself. This is in contrast to the endosteal implant, which is attached into the jawbone itself.

The sub-periosteal implant has small metal posts on it that the replacement teeth attach to. This special type of implant ends up integrating with the top surface of the natural bone it rests on and this is how it allows for stability of the new replacement teeth. Each implant is customized to the person who needs it. The procedure does not require advanced bone grafting like conventional methods of treatment. Newer 3-D technologies can also be applied to speed up the treatment process for this technique.

These types of implants are good for those who can't have any form of traditional implants because they have lost too much bone in their jaw, including the upper jaw. About 85% of these implants are placed in the mandible that has no teeth. The mandible is the lower part of the jaw.

Just thought I'd write you a few lines to let you know how happy and pleased I am with the subperiosteal implant Dr. Holtan did for me. Prior to the implant, I had four partial dentures made for me, over several years and not one of them was any good. As a result, my gum and jawbone shrank, the dentures didn't fit right when I would eat.

Now I can eat steak, pork chops, corn on the cob, nuts, food that I have not been able to eat for a long, long time. But aside from eating, which I enjoy so much, is that I look and feel better. All I can say is thank you Dr. Holtan for the great job you did. Thank for being so kind, considerate and thoughtful.

– Mildred K., Fort Myers, FL

This technique is rarely needed in today's world with the advancements in place at Dr. Holtan's. With that being said, for those patients where no other solutions exist, we still make it available so that no patient has to go without the hope of more solid teeth again for function, comfort, and feeling secure with solid teeth in public again. Few practices in North America are capable of utilizing this technique in these special circumstances, and we are pleased to be one of them.

Mini Dental Implants

Mini dental implants are very small diameter implants. Diameter refers to the side to side dimensions of the implant itself. A very small opening is placed that does not require cutting of the gum tissue, and a denture or teeth are anchored onto the mini implant. Mini dental implants are threaded into the bone much like a screw into a piece of wood and are immediately usable. Of course, by their very nature, they are minimally invasive, and no sutures or stitches are needed.

The fact is that patients really don't want invasive techniques. They don't want to spend a lot of time in the dentist's chair. Mini dental implants, according to Dr. Todd Shatkin, founder of the technique, have a success rate of 98% when used under the right circumstances and for the right patients. There's no down time after the procedure and very little pain.

Mini dental implants are approved by the FDA. Loose upper and lower dentures can be more stable when mini dental implants are used, and they are also perfect for replacing very specific types of missing teeth.

The most likely use for this type of special implant is for the cosmetic denture patient who would like a small increase in the retention of their denture.

Like other implant procedures, there's a network of dentists nationwide who understand this procedure – and that includes us at the dental office of Dr. Holtan. At your consultation, we can determine whether or not these mini dental implants will work for your particular situation and specific needs.

Cosmetic Single Front Implant Teeth

To understand the value and the challenge with missing front teeth visible in the smile, we must first discuss what makes a smile pleasing. A smile as seen in the mirror and from the viewer's perspective should be horizontally symmetrical – as if the teeth and gums are perfect mirror images of each other. When the teeth are symmetrical, the face looks balanced and is esthetically appealing. It also looks more youthful. Whenever this balance is off or uneven, the eye is drawn to the difference.

When you are young, it's also expected that your teeth will be more prominent in your smile. Researchers have even measured how much of the front teeth should show! They report that the average maxillary incisor display with the lips at rest is 1.91 mm in men and 3.4 mm in women. Patients with short upper lips and younger patients generally display more front teeth, which may be up to 3.65 mm. While a few millimeters don't sound like much, our eyes are amazingly good at picking up the tiniest details. If one's smile or gums are off by even several tenths of millimeters, other people will notice. Not only will they notice but you will too.

A missing tooth in the front such as one of the front teeth or eye teeth disrupts the perception of natural beauty in the face. When an implant is used in this location, and done properly, the face immediately regains its natural beauty.

Replacement of a single missing front tooth can be, and often is, one of the most challenging and costly types of implant dentistry. In many cases, other front teeth and even the gums may need cosmetic dentistry so that the balance and symmetry is returned to a pleasing state or simply maintained. It is vitally important to perform computerized simulations that look at gum, bone, and teeth in the front. This includes digital photographic plus 3-D analysis to properly determine the correct treatment course of action. No treatment step should be performed without these steps!

Based on observations and attendance at major educational meetings discussing this type of challenging situation, most dentists, even many of them professing expertise at dental implants, greatly underestimate how much is involved with recreating a natural appearance using dental implants visible in the smile. That underestimation can, and often does, lead to unwanted surprises for patients.

Oftentimes, it may take multiple grafts and multiple healing teeth (temporary crowns) to both contour the gum and bone to produce a result that is naturally undetectable by others. If your dentist makes this procedure sound simple or "easy" we suggest you immediately obtain a second or even a third opinion!

This covers the most basic "must knows" about dental implants. Needless to say, it's important that any dentist you are considering be well versed in each in order to develop an option that matches your situation and specific wants and needs.

Chapter 5
Have You Been Told You Can't Have a Dental Implant?

Do You Think You'll Suffer with Dentures Forever? You Can't Wear Dentures Another Day? You Can't Smile and Chew Like You Used To?

Right here in **Southwest Florida**, we have a complete approach to replacing lost or failing teeth that really works. That's why we are so deeply concerned when we see people who honestly want to smile confidently, chew confidently, look younger, and be healthier; people who are bitterly disappointed with their old dentures, partials, or failing teeth, who despair over earlier failed attempts to get their teeth straight.

Dental Implants Restore Lost Chewing Ability, Improve Appearance, End Embarrassment, and Give You Real

Self-Confidence. They are a Real Breakthrough.

Today dental implants are the profession's preferred method of replacing missing teeth. Because of proven success, preservation of existing teeth, and no susceptibility to dental decay (cavities), dental implants are the <u>answer</u> to missing teeth.

If you have been told you aren't a candidate because of a lack of supporting bone, you should come in and see us! We can almost always figure out ways to solve that problem so you can have implant restorations with today's news techniques or combinations of techniques that best fit your specific situation.

Let me tell you what I had before. I had a lot of sensitivity and a lot of gum disease, and my teeth weren't very nice looking. They were okay, but not great. They are beautiful now. I don't have any sensitivity; I can eat whatever I want. They are just wonderful!!

Actually, my gums have gotten better since I did all this. I had been told that I would need skin grafts and things like that, but now that is not even in the picture. My friends all want my teeth. I tell them to come to you and get them. Thank you. I love them.

Are You Embarrassed to Smile or Open Your Mouth Because of Missing Teeth, Unattractive Replacements, or Ill-Fitting Dentures or Partials?

Scientists at the University of Wisconsin School of Medicine and Public Health report that more than 35 million Americans have lost all their teeth and 178 million have lost at least one tooth. Most are unaware of what dentistry can do to improve their health. Implants can restore your chewing function to the equivalent of someone with natural teeth.

What Happened When They Lost Their Dentures?

During the Great East Japan Earthquake in March 2011, many older victims lost their removable dentures. Three to five months later, a survey was done with 715 denture wearers in the area. One hundred twenty-three of them had lost their dentures and **these people showed a significantly higher relative risk** for eating difficulties, speech problems, embarrassment with smiling, laughing or showing their teeth, emotional distress, and problems related to social interaction. These changes happened very quickly.

It's bad enough to have gone through an earthquake; just imagine how bad it would be to go through that disaster PLUS not have teeth in the rush to try to return to a normal life after the trauma! This was the first time a study like this had been conducted and the results were shocking. ***Even more shocking, almost no dentists*** outside of Japan paid attention to any of this information, **but we did**.

The bottom line of the study was direct proof that denture loss impairs eating and speaking ability, thus discouraging communication with others, which leads to all manner of negative social changes. The changes were much faster than any U.S., Canadian, European, or U.K. dentist would guess!

What have you been putting up with for months or even years since you lost one or more teeth? Ultimately the same social and mental health affects results, although, unlike in the Japanese survivors' cases, it's likely happened gradually and with little notice as you changed your behavior and routines.

Do You Suffer from These Effects of Missing and Failing Teeth?

- ✓ Pain on chewing
- ✓ Anxiety about your smile
- ✓ Avoid eating in public
- ✓ Ill-fitting/unattractive partials
- ✓ Nutritional disorders
- ✓ Teeth are unsightly
- ✓ Avoid certain foods
- ✓ Teeth are uncomfortable
- ✓ Teeth do not look real
- ✓ Teeth grinding
- ✓ Difficulty in dealing with stress
- ✓ Social embarrassment
- ✓ Difficulty in sleeping
- ✓ Difficulty swallowing
- ✓ Change in foods you eat
- ✓ Face falling in
- ✓ Altered taste of food
- ✓ Inconvenience
- ✓ Loss of support for the face

- ✓ Shrinking bone
- ✓ Gag reflex
- ✓ A need to feel whole again
- ✓ Bad breath that won't go away
- ✓ Feel older than you are
- ✓ Loss of self-esteem
- ✓ Depression over your teeth
- ✓ Unattractive smile
- ✓ Difficulty chewing
- ✓ Mouth sores
- ✓ Difficulty speaking
- ✓ Unstable dentures
- ✓ Burning sensations
- ✓ Unnatural feel
- ✓ Increased wrinkles
- ✓ Ashamed to smile
- ✓ Digestive disorders
- ✓ Shrinking gums
- ✓ Headaches
- ✓ Must use denture adhesive
- ✓ Jaw is sore
- ✓ Numbness in face and lips

- ✓ Withdrawal from social interaction
- ✓ Difficulty in dating relationships or sex life because of your teeth
- ✓ Limitations of foods that can be eaten/restricted diet
- ✓ Difficulty adjusting to life without your own teeth
- ✓ Food trapped between or under your teeth
- ✓ Avoid being seen in public
- ✓ Depressed/insecure without my partials/dentures
- ✓ Denture teeth move so much I don't wear them
- ✓ Avoid foods I would like to have
- ✓ I chew better *without* my partials/dentures

New Research Shows Connection

Between Tooth Loss and Slowing Mind

Yes, it's a very long list of things that ultimately can happen when teeth are missing, or when you are putting up with 18th century denture appliances, or when you are in the process of losing teeth. Now that you know how missing teeth are affecting you, it's good to find out what others have experienced, too.

How scientists ever decided to measure walking speed of those with teeth versus those with no teeth is surely a story unto itself, and that's exactly what they did at the University College in London. This new study was recently published in the *Journal of the American Geriatrics Society*. It was no small study either, as the researchers examined the walking speed and memory of 3,166 adults who were 60 and over.

Of course, they had to consider the fact that some of the study volunteers had existing health problems, drinking or smoking issues, or were depressed. And others tended to move slow perhaps due to their socioeconomic status. But in the end the truth came out – *those who had lost all their natural teeth and had a poor memory were worse 10 years later both in mental state and physical ability to walk.*

Just one more reason on a very long list of reasons on why it's so incredibly important to maintain the ability to chew as we age.

More Blunt Truth About
Missing Teeth

Missing Teeth Biologically Impair Man

Man is the _only_ animal that can live without any teeth. But how well?!

Only the ignorant would fail to recognize the implication of this: *missing teeth undoubtedly hampers any human being in such a state, making it more difficult biologically to function.*

You Will Need Your Teeth Longer

Man is living longer. The average age of lifespan continues to lengthen. At the time of Alexander the Great (356-323 BC) the average lifespan was 21 years! Scientists are now predicting 150-year lifespans within the next 15 to 50 years. People are living longer. They need their teeth longer – *YOU **will need your teeth longer***.

Missing Teeth Help Destroy Self-Confidence and Change How You Smile

(Do You Hide Your Smile?)

It is readily apparent when a front tooth is missing. It is a big deal, and everybody knows it. But what about the teeth on the side that are missing? Some people kid themselves into thinking it doesn't show.

Do you hold your lips a certain way...so no one can see your "hole?" Do you turn away from people...even if only slightly to mask the "gap"?

Do you restrict your smile from a big grin even at the funniest moments?

A Single Missing Tooth Can Cause Damage

That You Can't Feel or See Until It Is Often Too Late

Just one. That's right – <u>ONE</u>. One tooth missing can lead to the same cascade of events that has caused millions of people to lose other teeth needlessly.

It is the missing tooth that doesn't show, or only shows a little bit, that people kid themselves into thinking "everything is okay." It isn't. Few, if any, people would dream of leaving a gap in the front of their mouth...visibly ruining their smile. But many will do it in the back of their mouth – which, even a missing tooth in the back, can eventually harm smile and health.

Yes, a missing tooth in the back can affect your smile and it often happens so slowly that you hardly notice until it becomes a major problem – costing more in dollars and time to fix? It could have been prevented.

Are You Making This Mistake?

Here is the mistake we don't want you to make: You say to yourself, "I can't see it, it doesn't hurt, I'll leave it like that." These are the words of the average, unknowing person who doesn't realize the serious and even life-threatening effects that loss of a tooth can cause.

Let's examine why: Mother Nature designed your teeth to work together, each tooth designed to perform a certain function. When a member of the group is lost, more work is required out of the remaining teeth.

The other teeth start to shift toward the hole left by the missing tooth. The teeth on either side tilt into the space; the tooth above grows down. Front teeth begin to shift and change as well and suddenly the visible teeth that everyone else sees are noticeably changing and one's smile begins to deteriorate.

Gaps open up. Teeth shift!

Your smile changes for the worse.

Now your **bite is thrown off**, almost always causing something called a "destructive bite." A destructive bite is one in which the way the teeth fit together when chewing causes damage simply by the incorrect fit between the chewing surfaces.

Destructive bites can cause **headaches**, **... jaw joint pain** that can be ***intolerable***, ... **broken teeth**, ... *and teeth that wear too fast*; in fact, a destructive bite will double the age of your teeth in just a few years.

Have you ever seen someone with short front teeth? Chances are about 20 to 1 that a destructive bite is the cause. Destructive bites ruin smiles. Don't let this happen to you.

Back to our missing tooth. The tooth that grows down into the space is now *threatened by gum disease* because of its awkward, poor position. The space where the missing tooth was creates a trap for food and bacteria that gives you an absolute fit trying to keep clean. **Gum disease is an infection that impacts the entire body, <u>doubling the risk for heart disease, heart attack</u>, and <u>multiple other health-related problems</u>.**

So literally, what was once "just a missing tooth" in the back can now be life threatening.

And, if one tooth missing can cause this many problems, *multiple missing teeth can cripple you.*

Missing teeth change the way you chew for the worse…your comfort in chewing diminishes, sometimes so severely that eating becomes a pain…a pain you are forced to live with every day of your life…a pain that doesn't get better by itself…a pain that only gets worse.

The more teeth you have missing, the worse it is and the faster a destructive bite can arise and lead to this downward spiral.

Diseased Teeth and Gums Threaten Your Health … (AND YOUR FAMILY'S HEALTH!)

Some people hold on to teeth that are diseased because they don't want to lose them; something very understandable. But because they are diseased and should be removed, they threaten their own health and, worse, the health of the ones they love the most! These same bacteria are infectious to others around you. You read this right; gum infections are infections to others!

An explanation: The bacteria on your teeth and in your gums travel to other parts of the body, wreaking havoc along the way such as:

o Heart disease is worsened

o Heart attack risks are increased up to 200%

o Stroke risks are increased

o Worsened arthritis

o Increased low birth weight in babies

o Pre-disposes you to illness generally

o Generalized decreased energy to cope with life

o Worsened diabetic conditions – more difficult to control and maintain

Those with gum infections are estimated to live 6-10 years less than those with healthy mouths!

We know...it is this bad. But more research is being done in this field. **It is likely that the effects of oral disease are far more dangerous than we presently know.**

Now here is the real kicker: <u>Those with diseased teeth and gums can and do spread these bacteria to their spouses, children, and family members</u>.

Who doesn't share a spoon or glass or bit of food? According to some studies the chances are about 70% that people who live together will "share" the same bacteria. Who hasn't experienced one member of the family getting the flu and subsequently everyone else in the family does, too?

All the more reason that every family member should work to attain and maintain dental health. It is *the right thing to do*. No sane person wants to contaminate his spouse and or children and harm their health.

Dear Dr. Holtan,

Now that the work on my lower implants is completed, it is with a great deal of enthusiasm I write this letter of thanks for the excellent work you did. They look and feel like my natural teeth which I was hoping for but did not believe was really possible.

It was surprising to me to find the whole procedure virtually painless. Being "a confirmed coward" when pain is involved, I had psyched myself up to facing a horrendously painful ordeal. Thankfully, this never occurred. No doubt, they would be painful procedures were done while I was under sedation. The swelling of my jaws afterwards was not painful, just inconvenient for 3 or 4 days.

If at any time you should have a "Doubting Thomas" among your potential implant recipients, I will be happy to answer any questions he or she might have – from an "implant" point of view, or the "horse's mouth," so to speak.

– Helen M., Cape Coral, FL

Chapter 6
Do You Love to Eat?

Why Enjoying the Taste and Experience of Your Food Is More Important than Ever

Eating is one of life's pleasures…the foods we eat fill our senses…just the sight of a beautifully prepared meal can make one's mouth water in excited anticipation…the sweet aroma can bring those you love rushing to the table …the feel of foods in your fingers and in your mouth amplifies the experience of the pleasure of eating...the sound of laughter and congenial conversation fills dinner tables throughout the world.

And of course, the taste of your food…Ahhhhh…the taste…the tangy orange...the tart lemon…the salty potato chip...the sizzling steak right off the grill...the crisp apple…the crunchy raw carrot…the hard cashew and the soft banana...the sweet chocolate… All of these are part of the food experience that most all of us relish.

Mealtimes are when we all join together and enjoy not only the foods but also

the relationships of family, friends, and all the special someones who make life worth living. Our meals are times we unite with those we care about and put aside the stresses of the day.

It is a rejuvenation of not only our bodies with needed nutrients...and a rejuvenation of our relationship with those we value...with those who add richness to our lives.

Knowing how important these times are to your health and happiness makes having *teeth that look good, feel good, and function properly that much more vital to quality living every day of your life*. Many of our patients going through life-changing implant treatment are surprised by what they had given up with their family and friends and interactions, *especially* around the dining room table.

Dentures Decrease Chewing Ability and Function and Change the Foods You Eat for the Worse

Dentures and partial dentures take the pleasure out of food and negatively impact one's ability to enjoy the simple pleasures of mealtime with family and friends. There are very good reasons why dentures and partials fail you and why you can't chew comfortably and smile confidently no matter how hard you try with these archaic devices.

Natural teeth with their roots implanted in the gum and surrounded by bone are able to exert up to 250 pounds per square inch of chewing pressure. For normal chewing, natural teeth exert an average pressure of 45 pounds per square inch of force, ranging up to 75 pounds.

• With dentures, the average chewing pressure is reduced to 14 pounds per square inch and, for some wearers, as little as 5 pounds per square inch. THIS IS A 5- to 15-FOLD DECREASE IN CHEWING EFFECTIVENESS! Is it any wonder these devices are a letdown? Is it a surprise that less than 1 in 20 denture wearers, especially those who have had "traditional denture" therapy, report being satisfied with their denture?

• If you are a denture wearer, you know or have found that this tremendous loss of pressure means having to completely change your eating habits. Many foods need to be eliminated completely. You have to cut your food into small pieces.

• The average lower denture shifts side to side approximately ½ inch during chewing and is one of the problems that make getting used to it so difficult. This same shifting is the reason that most denture wearers don't wear the lower denture unless absolutely necessary – such as when they go out in public.

The types of food that are easier to chew are soft carbohydrates and other high-calorie foods because of their softness. Therefore, denture wearers often fall into two categories: overweight, because of all the calories, and at the other extreme, underweight – because of the inability to chew food correctly. This alteration of the diet can cause a tipping point in general health and contribute to other major medical problems.

• Denture wearers also complain that the **taste, temperature, texture, and enjoyment of food are decreased**. They may add additional salt and spices to food to give it more taste.

• It's not really surprising that this occurs because the plastic of their dentures insulates the tissue that is responsible for giving a person "the sense" of their food. **The result of increased weight and excess salt can lead to high blood pressure and problems of the digestive tract**. Forty percent (40%) of heart disease is related to high blood pressure and arteriosclerosis.

• According to Dr. Carl Misch, who was one of the world's most renowned implant pioneers, **the average denture wearer has a 10-year shorter lifespan!**

The Whole-Body Health and Teeth Connection

Speaking of health, there's quite a connection between what is happening in the mouth and your overall health. You might already know about the connection of health with gum disease since news reports began talking about it about five years ago. Gum disease is the #1 cause of tooth loss, but the story of what's important to your whole beyond just tooth loss is even more important to understand.

Here are just a few of the things that news anchors have reported:

✓ People with gum disease are 40% more likely to have a chronic disease, including heart disease.

✓ Up to 91% of patients with heart disease have periodontal disease, but in the general population, only 66% of people have it.

In fact, the infections in the mouth around the gum line have been linked to bad bacteria that even set up little pimple-like infections in the arteries and contributed to plaque build-up that narrows arteries and affects blood flow. This inflammation in the mouth is linked to inflammation in one's blood vessels!

We all tend to think of arterial plaque that causes "hardening of the arteries" as a thick layer that covers all the blood vessels in the body. This is far from the truth, except maybe in severe hardening of the arteries. That's what the American Society of Microbiology says. Once the bacteria from the mouth or other infections in the body find a minute tear in an artery, they attach themselves in that artery. The body – in all its glory – comes to the rescue and then tries to send in the immune system army to clean it up. This response is good in that it contains infections, but it also causes collateral damage due to the inflammation. Dental gum inflammation unnecessarily keeps our inflammatory response at a higher "alert" level than necessary.

The problem is that inflammation attracts all types of white blood cells to the area, and it's almost like building a mud cake in the artery. There's a good chance that the mud cake will only get bigger if the infection continues – or if there is a lot of inflammation elsewhere in the body that the immune system has to fight.

The process continues and then before you know it, the "mud cake" in the artery is now blocking the blood vessel 75 or 95%!

Check Your Tongue for Bacteria Right Now!

And here's a big tip for you and your whole family: Have you seen those tongue cleaners at the store? The bacteria in your mouth is not only found on the teeth and gum but 50% of it is on the tongue!

Stick out your tongue and go to the mirror and look. Do you see a coating of white or dark on top of your tongue? This is a mixture of bacteria, fungi, yeast like Candida, and byproducts from infections. This coating is contributing to tooth loss just as much as the bacteria around your gums because it's feeding the bacteria around your gums. The acidic products of the bacteria can also eat away at the gums and the tooth structure leading to dental decay. When the teeth start getting wobbly and loose, it means that loss of the bony support around the teeth is well underway.

By the way, archaeologists found tongue cleaners that date back to 100 A.D. They are convinced that royalty and nobility also cleansed their tongues daily, so this isn't some type of fad.

Diabetics CAN Save Their Teeth!

If you're a diabetic, you hopefully know all about periodontal disease and how it affects your blood sugar levels. Infections in the body of a diabetic cause higher blood sugar levels even though the person doesn't usually want to eat when they have an infection. The inflammation from the infection affects the body's ability to use insulin. Gum infections also make it more difficult to regulate blood sugar levels in diabetics. Physicians are just now being educated about this link between gum infections and difficulty in managing diabetes.

What you may be figuring out here is that you do have quite a bit of control over tooth loss in the first place – but only after you know these facts. If you stop eating sugar and clean your teeth more regularly, your health could actually improve.

For the diabetic, the benefit is even greater. Yes, not only can eliminating harmful bacteria through brushing, flossing, tongue cleaning, and professional dental cleanings prevent decay and tooth loss, but by doing so you can also positively influence the management of diabetic problems and reduce the use of medications for disease management!

Infections in the Mouth Make Other Diseases Worse

It's not only heart disease that is connected with infections in the mouth. Chalk up one point for rheumatoid arthritis and another for obesity. Rheumatoid arthritics have less pain when they clean up their mouth of infections. Obesity is interesting because the extra fat in the body around the middle sends out signals to the rest of the body to increase inflammation. The white blood cell army is then activated and hits all the spots in the body where there might only be a slight infection, magnifying it.

Pneumonia and lung problems such as COPD have the same response – the worse the periodontal disease, the worse the lung problems get. The body can only fight so many infections at one time!

Consider Changing Your Oral Hygiene Habits TODAY!

To start, brush your teeth after every meal and not simply with a toothbrush but with a

Sonicare electric toothbrush. The Sonicare electric toothbrush rocks! Why? Because it can almost eliminate the need for flossing! If you don't floss, do yourself and your teeth and gums a favor: buy the most basic Sonicare model without all the bells and whistles and use it 2-3 times each day.

Next, if you can get in the habit of flossing, floss at least daily. If you have spaces between the teeth, then there are variety of other cleaning devices that will help you keep the spaces clean. For those who want to skip flossing, either a WaterPik or a "shower floss" device used on a daily basis are the routes to go. Both can be found by searching online at Amazon.com.

Finally, start scraping your tongue with a tongue scraper. This process physically removes millions of bacteria that can contribute to tooth loss. Before long, your tongue will even look a lot better. Your breath will be fresher. And your food will taste better. You'll find these scrapers in the drugstore in the dental section or online at Amazon.com.

There's also a type of tongue cleaner that is clinically proven by dentists at the University of Buffalo, UCLA Fresh Breath Clinic, and University of Minnesota. It's called the

OOLITT Tongue Cleaner. Believe it or not, it was patented over 20 years ago. Where have we all been that we never heard about this important tool that deserves room right next to our toothbrush?

If you follow these simple rules mentioned above for oral health, you could save any number of teeth for the long term. These protocols along with professional help from a competent dental hygienist can mean greatly lowering the general health risks that stem from inflammation starting with the gums. So do take them seriously!

Dear Dr. Holtan,

I feel and look years younger with my new dentures. My face is now filled out and have gotten rid of that "sunken in look." Thank you, thank you. I have worn plates for years and was getting older looking each day, you have made me smile again. You can count on me to be your best advertisement ever.

– Trudie W., Cleveland, OH

Chapter 7
Don't Let Missing Teeth Rob You of the Pleasures of Living

Who wants to cut his food up into baby-sized pieces in order to cope with "getting it down"? It's too embarrassing. Who wants to bite into their food and realize this normal-sized piece is just way too big to manage? Spitting into a napkin is never fun!!!

Some people try to cope with their lack of chewing ability by swallowing foods almost whole! **This alone can be life threatening**. People die from choking every day. Assuming the un-chewed chunk doesn't <u>choke you</u>, it **gives your digestive tract fits**: *constipation and irregularity* and "who knows what else."

So, what is the other choice? Give up the foods you like to eat that provide the nutrients you need… If you can't chew your food, change your diet to soft foods… You are reduced to foods that have the same consistency as baby food. You know a steak just doesn't seem the same after going through a blender!

Implants Help −A Lot!!

Studies indicate that after 2 months of having implanted-supported replacement teeth, patients were able to increase their maximal biting force by 85%. After 3 years the average chewing force increased **300% compared to before implant treatment!**

Overall, the <u>chewing ability of patients</u> with <u>implant-supported teeth is roughly equal to patients</u> with healthy, natural teeth, and vastly superior to patients with conventional dentures.

Missing Teeth Encourage Wrinkling and Premature Aging

The bone that surrounds the teeth must be stimulated from within or the body dissolves (resorbs) it. This results in dentures or partials that repeatedly need to be relined or remade. It also creates and worsens *creases and wrinkles in the face*.

The distance as measured between the tip of the nose and the tip of chin decreases. The nose then appears larger or more prominent. The face begins to look like it is frowning when at rest because the corners of the mouth pull down and form creases. The lower part of the face looks fallen or sunken in. The chin looks like it comes to a point or a "witch's chin." It is this collapsed middle 1/3 that makes one look truly old.

From Dr. Holtan:

I learned about the effect these changes could have on a person long before becoming a dentist. One of my mom's friends had lost a significant number of her teeth and felt so "ugly" that she got to the point where she wouldn't leave the house. It all came to a head one day when she was in the laundromat.

She had been feeling bad and had even stated "I look like a witch!" when she was over for some coffee. She was about in tears and I could see the desperation in her tone of voice and in her mannerisms. She felt robbed of her life. She wanted to open up a business to save animals from "death row" at the local animal shelter, and had all these noble plans in life, yet she felt blocked – like she couldn't progress forward looking like she did.

And then all it took was one small child in the laundromat to put her over the edge. "Are you a witch?" he asked her.

Well, you can't really blame the little kid for saying what was on his mind. He probably had been reading some series of story books and was curious. Maybe he secretly hoped that

she was and could give her some direction...
Who knows what was really going on in that
small boy's mind?

"No, I'm not a witch," she said to the
boy. "Do I look like one?"

"Yeah, kind of...," he said back and then
scurried away.

She had to be counseled by my mom for
several days after that incident, and when my
mom asked her to go on a trip with some other
women, this lady said, "No way! I'm not going
anywhere until I get my teeth fixed."

Imagine the emotional chaos she had to
experience at that time – and all because she
needed dental implants at a time when they
were not available to her. Today her story and
life would have been far different. No patient
today needs to go through this!

Missing teeth affect the face in other
ways. Jowls may form and make the face look
unnatural. The tongue may actually enlarge
because of the increased demands placed on it
from missing teeth. This can cause speech and
chewing problems. Thankfully, the tongue
adapts well to implant-supported replacement
teeth.

No wonder dentures may affect a person's health, both physically and psychologically. A sense of security may be lost. It may affect success in personal or business relationships. It may alter your speech, looks, and function.

Many a patient has come in looking older than their chronological age (a 50-year-old who looks 70, for example). After dental implants they enjoy **dental and facial rejuvenation**. Often the change makes them look 10-15 years younger than their actual age. Moreover, those who receive treatment with implants slow down the clock of aging substantially. They **look younger longer**.

Warning!! If You're Considering Facial Plastic Surgery, Don't Make This Mistake!

If you are considering a "facelift" procedure of any kind, it's critically important to fix worn down teeth or replace missing teeth first! This will reset the correct proportions of the lower one-third of the face. If this step is skipped it reduces the results of even the best plastic surgeons! Unfortunately, most plastic surgeons don't realize the impact of this nor recommend a dental consultation before surgery is performed.

By fixing your teeth first, your surgery will not only have a better chance of success, but the results are likely to last longer since the surgeon won't be fighting the changes that the underlying teeth and bone have played in appearance.

Partial Dentures Cause Bone Loss, Too!

At the end of 5 years, only 40% of partial denture wearers are still wearing the partial denture made for them. Those patients still wearing partial dentures are all losing bone! What is the use and value of that?

• Of those wearing a partial, 50% chew better without it!

• In one study, after 8 years, 40% of teeth that hook to the partial were lost through decay or fracture. Yes, this means that a device still being prescribed by a significant percentage of dentists is literally an "extraction device!" If a dentist is recommending a partial denture to you, seek a consultation elsewhere!

• Partials exert pressure on the gum and bone, causing bone loss, which makes the partial even more difficult to wear.

Don't Hold onto Diseased Teeth Too Long Just to Save Your Teeth While Destroying Your Jaw Bones!

Gum and bone infections (periodontal disease) are a very destructive process that not only causes loss of teeth but also the remaining bone. Many people as a result of their deep desire to keep their teeth and to avoid dentures <u>are suffering with severely diseased teeth</u>.

The damage caused by this disease is often extensive and permanent. This causes severe loss of bone that could have been used for your implants!

It is possible that these teeth can be removed and for you to have a complete restoration of function without full dentures. Sometimes it is possible to treat some of these teeth and incorporate them, along with implants, into a fixed, non-removable full set of teeth. Ultimately, it takes a Type 3 Expert Level dentist, as we will discuss later in the guidebook, to help you navigate your choices.

If you feel you want to maintain your teeth, no matter how great the degree your gum problem currently is, it is still vitally important to have a consultation. Newer laser procedures (virtually painless!) allow us to halt gum infections and to stabilize remaining bone.

Again, when the gum infection is left untreated or is treated with conventional dental techniques or traditional periodontal "scaling and root planning" or "traditional periodontal surgery," the disease might be slowed but in many patients bone will still gradually dissolve away, making future treatment options more costly and complicated. With these new lasers we can kill the most harmful bacteria, stabilize your gums, and give you the longest amount of time with your natural teeth before moving to a permanent implant solution.

Denture Adhesives Are Not a Good Solution

In the United States each year more than $90 million is spent by the public on denture adhesives. The denture adhesives themselves have unpleasant tastes, must be reapplied often, give an inconsistent fit of the denture, have continued costs, and create embarrassing circumstances. The adhesives also lead to overgrowths of harmful bacteria and yeasts and act as the adhesive acts as an incubator in the warm and moist oral environment.

It's no surprise that most patients refer to these adhesives as denture "goop" because of the sticky and un-tasty mess it leaves both inside the denture and stuck to delicate gum tissues. It routinely shows up as one of the top things denture patients hate about traditional dentures.

89% Better Outlook on Life

For many people in our culture the loss of teeth is associated with aging. Implants give a **psychological lift to these people with missing teeth who would otherwise have some feelings of inadequacy related to aging and loss of teeth.**

In fact, a study by Branemark, a global leader in implants and the maker of the specialized All-on-4 implant, reported that 89% of patients treated with dental implants judged their psychological health improved compared to before treatment. The majority of these patients perceived their implant supported replacement teeth as an integral part of their own body.

Dental Implants Give Predictable Success – Far Better Than Traditional Fixed Bridges

Several studies have been published that indicate that implant treatment of the patient with missing teeth is more predictable long term than many other more typical therapies in dentistry, including the often used 3-tooth fixed bridge.

The success rate for 3-tooth bridges on natural teeth is about 85% over a 5-year period. For implant-supported teeth the success rate is 90% or more for the same period of time. Now, while those short-term success rates are pretty similar, once we leave the 5-year period something interesting starts to happen. As time marches on, the bridges begin to fail because of either decay or because of a fracture of one of the natural teeth supporting the appliance. In a bit, we'll go more into detail about both issues.

The way a dental bridge works is that the natural teeth immediately on each side of a space where natural teeth are missing are "mowed down" to small nubs and the nubs are used as support for the appliance to rest upon. The middle section, replacing the missing tooth or teeth, is suspended out from these supports on the natural teeth. This is why it is called a bridge," since it crosses an empty space and rests on something firm at both ends.

No matter how great of a bridge technique the dentist has or how great the actual bridge device, all bridges exert extra stress on the natural teeth they are attached to and ultimately damage those natural teeth. The longer the bridge span, meaning the more missing teeth the middle part replaces, the more likely it is that the dentist will have had to "mow down" even more natural teeth to support the two ends. Needless to say, this not only damages more teeth but a longer middle part puts added stress onto the natural teeth at the ends.

As time goes by, everyday chewing causes the glue holding the bridge to chip away and bacteria begin to collect around the natural teeth. Decay then forms and either a repair has to be made or a root canal has to be performed because the decay silently spreads deep into the teeth damaged by the original procedure. Next thing you know the bridge needs to be replaced and more natural teeth are now "mowed down."

Beyond decay, another way bridges begin to fail after the 5-year mark is that the roots of the natural teeth bearing all the extra stress that they were not designed for fracture and then a tooth is lost.

Ultimately, no matter how we look at this device, in most patients over the course of time a cycle of more treatment and more extractions is all a part of the game of "dental bridge." Additionally, the long-term cost is high because of the never-ending redoing of the dental work!

Currently, the most ethical and educated (the Type #3 Expert Level Dentist) will no longer recommend this device to any patient because of all of the issues put forth above, and we are certainly in that crowd of the most informed dentists on this subject. We believe a time is coming in the near future where the performance of this procedure would be malpractice.

So, what about dental implants? Well, after the 5-year mark, dental implants filling empty spaces, instead of a traditional bridge procedure, have basically the same success rate of 90% or greater and there is no damage to other teeth and a lower chance of additional tooth loss! Eventually both the partial denture and the traditional bridge will no longer be on any dentist's menu of services. Since many dentists still don't know the above numbers by heart, if a dentist is recommending either of these devices to you, it's time to get a second opinion!

Beyond those numbers showing just how successful implants are as compared to bridges, here is another. A study by Branemark, the inventor of modern dental implants, reported a 93% success rate over the last 10 years for the subperiosteal implant (a particular implant type that sits on the bone under the gum). Turner and Small have scientifically reported success rates between 94% and 98% for the last 10 years.

All of these studies reported implant treatment for lower jaws with all missing teeth. This is particularly good news because the lower denture is the one that is the most problematic. Of course, success cannot be guaranteed, but it is nice to know that success rates are so high.

Our own success rates are now at 90+% at our dental offices

Dental Implants Work with a Single or Multiple Missing Teeth

Today we can replace single teeth, several teeth in a section of the jaw, or the entire arches of teeth. Dental implants allow you to go from the state of advanced gum disease with loose, uncomfortable, and infected teeth to a full set of non-removable teeth.

Every situation involving missing teeth presents its own set of unique requirements, and there are ways to meet almost every need. Your best course of action is to seek out an Expert Level Type 3 Dentist and have a consultation regarding your specific situation.

Almost All People with Missing Teeth

Can Benefit from Implants but...

Beware of Those Claiming a "One-Size/One-Treatment Plan Fits All" Situation!

It is rare that a person cannot receive an implant or a combination of implant types. There are also no two people alike in their need for dental reconstruction. and different needs for implants within the same jaw exists, too. Today we have available many types of implants designed to accommodate multiple problems.

The ability to utilize multiple implant techniques is an essential ingredient to the successful use of implants. **No one design will cover all situations.** Function, appearance, comfort, and inconvenience dictate implant selection.

There are several prominent corporate dental chains operating now that promise and "high-pressure, hard-sell" virtually every patient who walks in the door that their one single treatment option is the absolute best solution for everyone and every situation. This is like going into a local store of any kind and the store owner promising you that the one item they carry is the only thing you could possibly need. Where's the logic in that?!?

Again, each patient is too unique for such a cookie-cutter approach. If someone tells you there is nothing but one best option, once again, it's time to get a second opinion!

I cannot begin to tell you how pleased I am with Dr. Holtan and his entire staff. Dr. Holtan is very well educated, explained in detail, as much as I wanted, the procedure, process and costs.

I had gone to other highly recommended dentists for their estimate and review who perform the same procedure, and unquestionably, Dr. Holtan is superior and stands out well above all the rest.

I am probably the worst patient a dentist would want as I had many poor past experiences. Dr. Holtan and staff were always kind, assuring, answered all questions and, as importantly, made me feel very comfortable and confident before, during and after the procedure.

Due to my many fears and apprehensions, I waited at least 5 years to have this procedure done. How I wish I had this procedure done several years ago by Dr. Holtan. You are doing yourself a huge injustice if you do not see Dr. Holtan before making a final decision. He is the best!

– Charles P., Naples, FL

Chapter 8
Advantages of Dr. Holtan's Method of Implant Dentistry

30 Advantages of Our Method of Implant Strategy

1) <u>Proven success</u> of dental implants for our patients.

2) Experienced know-how that solves your problems...using what works for you and your ***individual*** situation.

3) *Preservation of existing teeth*.

4) Rejuvenation of the form and shape of the face.

5) Improvement in the facial dimensions, especially the lower one-third of the face.

7) <u>Wrinkle reduction</u> in many cases. Often a dental facelift is a happy byproduct of dental implant treatment.

8) **<u>Gorgeous smiles.</u>**

9) An advanced "smart" system of diagnosis and treatment.

10) Restored <u>chewing ability</u>.

11) **<u>Relief</u>** from the pain of dentures and tooth-damaging partial dentures.

12) No embarrassing accidents of teeth falling out.

13) Enhanced **<u>zest for life (return of joie de vivre)</u>**.

14) Getting noticed by that special someone you want noticing you.

15) More smiles, a lot more smiles.

16) A system that carefully considers how to make your teeth look their best while *<u>functioning properly and staying healthy</u>*.

17) Built on a thoroughness approach that gives you predictable results.

18) **Stops your situation from getting worse.**

19) A physician of the mouth approach applying the science of comfort, health, function, and longevity to the teeth, gums, jaw joints, and chewing mechanism, based on solid principles...time tested and true...coupled with the latest dental research.

20) An investment in yourself that pays big dividends every day of your life.

21) A demanding discipline that is a daily challenge, but one that our teams and we fully embrace. We won't compromise results. We will give options but refuse to give a bad option. If we wouldn't offer or perform a given treatment on a loved one or close friend, you can be guaranteed it will not be offered to you!

22) A unified system that uses the *best of the best in techniques and technology.*

23) An ever-evolving system of care designed to get great treatment results, <u>enhance comfort</u>, and <u>reduce anxiety</u> and leave you with a <u>radiant smile</u>.

24) The result of an extended study of over 20 years that costs huge untold sums **and thousands of hours of additional training**

and research beyond what is required to be a dentist…that continues on even today.

25) *The end of Dental Embarrassment!*

26) A comprehensive approach combining the **best practices of treatment** learned and observed inside and outside the profession.

27) A system that carefully considers how to make your teeth look their best while functioning properly and staying healthy.

28) The artistic pursuit of beautiful teeth and gorgeous smiles.

29) Comfortable, confident chewing in social situations.

30) Preservation of your youthful appearance – resistance to aging.

If Dentistry Has Been Difficult for You, the Dread Is Gone! It's Over! You Can Relax!

Really you can. I know, I know. It can be hard for you if you have had a nightmare of an experience. But no longer because…

Stone Age Dentistry Is a Thing of the Past

Dentistry of just 20-30 years ago was absolutely Stone Age compared to dentistry today in our office. At Dr. Holtan's dental office, we recognize what has stopped so many from having a beautiful smile they are proud of and achieving real dental health for life.

And, we have done something about it. **Our system uses newly developed techniques and technology to make your visit easier, faster, and more comfortable.**

Thank you for everything. It is extremely rare to meet a person with a heart as giving as yours. Your kindness is really appreciated, thanks for everything.

– Naples Football Team, Naples, FL

The commitment to your comfort starts with a unique office design created to produce a noise-reducing, quiet environment.

The dental chairs themselves feature Swedish foam that comfortably molds to your body, making it easier to relax.

Even the colors were chosen scientifically to help create a relaxing environment.

We use CD players and stereo headphones so you can hear the sounds you want and drown out the sounds you don't!

We Are "Armed to The Teeth" with Technology and Techniques to Create a Better Dental Experience

We have an understanding of what the typical fearful or anxious patient experiences – and just how different it can be for them. If this describes you, you'll be comforted first by a special chair-side manner that puts you at ease.

Then there is the matter of getting numb. We use a unique, virtually painless numbing method that is easy to experience.

Dr. Holtan and everyone at the office are such talented and caring people. I can't express enough to all of you how fortunate I feel.

I am happy to have found you all. I feel confident and happy again. How can one ever repay you for giving me my smile back once again?

What a wonderful difference in my life...so happy! Thank you again for really helping me make one of the best decisions of my life.

The office manager instilled the confidence in trusting Dr. Holtan's talent and was she ever right about that!

– Pat S., Naples, FL

You'll be offered a blanket to keep you warm. Then, we'll give as brief or detailed explanation as <u>you</u> would like about what we find, what we do, and why. This full explanation helps you know what to expect.

For those needing something extra, that bit of extra help in managing themselves, we utilize oral sedation to take the "edge off." Typically, the pill given an hour before the procedure is triazolam, a drug that's in the same family as Valium. It makes you drowsy although you will still be conscious.

Sometimes a larger dose may be offered to put you in the state of moderate sedation, the state of consciousness where your words are slurred while speaking and you don't remember much of what is happening; many patients say they remember absolutely nothing about their visit. You may even fall asleep during the dental implant procedure, but tapping on your shoulder will most likely wake you.

If you choose oral sedation during your procedure, for safety, a friend or family member will need to drive you home. If you have traveled a distance to see us, our team will escort you to your local hotel and make sure you reach your room safely.

At the dental office of Dr. Holtan, you'll also receive a special type of local anesthetic in the area of your mouth where the implant will be that "deadens" sensations in the area so that you feel nothing during the implant procedure.

Even if you are stoic about pain, you will still be offered our full range of methods meant to make your experience virtually painless. If you are investigating these services in another part of the country, you have the right to ask your dentist for oral sedation. It's a well-accepted idea in the profession that if something can be done to make the patient more comfortable, it should be done. For complex procedures, if sedation services are not being offered it is a sign to seek out an opinion from another professional.

There are a lot of people for whom oral sedation has totally transformed their dental health – those who have very sensitive teeth, those who feel pain if you scratch them with your nail, those who have gag reflexes when their mouth is open and someone is poking around in it, and those who have hours and hours of dental work that needs to be accomplished.

Sedation dentistry may also include another option – medical anesthesia. We have a fully licensed anesthesiologist available who can attend to your comfort if necessary.

And just for the record, you might want to know that dentists often have to have a special permit/license to offer sedation dentistry to their patients. The state/province regulates this procedure.

Why not go to the dentist and not feel any pain? The technology is available for exactly that to happen. Like many other patients of Dr. Holtan, your dental implant appointment can be one of the best visits to the dentist you've ever had in your life!

I was referred to Dr. Holtan by a girlfriend of mine who is a patient of his. I came in as a new patient having spent many years dealing with periodontal disease and going through many different upper plates that never fit properly, and I was losing my teeth on the lower. I was told by a dentist and a periodontist that I didn't have enough bone support for implants, but this was not an obstacle for the All-on-Four.

The day of the surgery, I remember coming into the office, but I do not remember leaving. I woke up later on that night asking, "Do I have teeth in my mouth? Is everything finished?" I felt nothing at all, and it was all done! A little sore the next day, and a few days after, but nothing like I thought it would be.

Since the time I came into the office, the people, the staff, Dr. Holtan, everyone has been absolutely marvelous. As an All-on-Four patient, I would absolutely recommend this procedure to all denture wearers. I could not be happier with everything."

– Cathy

Chapter 9
Looking Good

The cosmetic question has never been better answered than it is today. Of course, the function has already been assured with the stability and retention given to replacement teeth by dental implants.

With the materials and techniques available today we are able to create a natural appearance. Lost lip and cheek support from the shrinkage of gums are managed well using implant techniques. Many times, when there has been a great deal of bone loss, lip and cheek support can be built right into the tooth portion of reconstruction, helping to fill out what is missing.

Dental implants also increase your ability to taste and savor food because of the fact that you can chew your food properly again and your taste buds can once again do their intended job, which is to sense how food tastes and its texture. Tastes and textures that were only memories return quickly after you get your teeth and implants.

Attractiveness Determines How Other People

Perceive and Treat You

Scientific research has proven what many people already know: **the better you look, the better others treat you.** The point here is that the advantage of attractiveness is very greatly *underestimated.* The size and reach of attractiveness are huge. Why? Because people who are seen as attractive are believed to be smarter, more talented, kinder, and more honest.

This is true throughout our entire society. In other words, your smile and teeth determine a great deal of how much other people want to be around you. With a great smile, you become more *promote-able*...more attractive to the opposite sex...more likely to be viewed as someone who others want to be friends with...more trustworthy.

Social Advantages of Looking Good

Good-looking people enjoy a tremendous social advantage. They are viewed as more intelligent. They are better liked. They are seen as having more desirable personalities. Attractive people are *more persuasive* and more likely to be given help by others.

An Investment in Yourself

Most people find the increased confidence provided by secure implant-supported teeth as well as improved appearance and vastly improved function more than offset the relatively minor discomfort and inconvenience associated with even the most complex implant procedures.

Implants Make Good Economic Sense

Admittedly, dental implants can be a significant investment. Before committing to any investment, you should always consider its amount, under what terms it could be paid, the quality of what you get in exchange, and what your alternatives are.

The initial investment of a dental implant can be higher than other methods of treatment. Dental implants can run from $3,700 for a single tooth to $22,000 per arch or more. Usually not every tooth requires replacement with a dental implant. Typically for denture sufferers, a dental implant resolution to this problem can range from $12,000 to $22,000.

Fees for this special, unique service <u>vary significantly</u> from individual to individual. Why? Because everyone is different. Just as each person has a different fingerprint, you have a different need than everyone else. This makes it impossible to quote a fee over the phone without examination. There isn't a one-size-fits-all service. Each need, want, and desire is just too variable, and matching these things to which option will best satisfy you can only be done with time spent together listening to your concerns. Most of our patients who had been to other practices offering similar services tell us that they almost never felt truly listened to and were glad they finally found a practice where *every concern expressed* was taken into account before recommending any treatment options.

If you find a practice quoting fees over the phone without seeing you live and in person, or if you find a practice recommending any type of treatment before they've seen you in person, or if you find a practice that only offers a "one size fits every patient's situation" option, be aware that they are doing a disservice to you and not fulfilling their professional obligation of understanding your individual needs as a patient. Under these circumstances, seek a second opinion.

Additionally, if a fee is quoted over the phone and it seems rather low, the old saying of "if it sounds too good to be true, then it probably is" is very likely at work. In fact, oftentimes when a low fee is quoted there are many additional "surprise" fees later that come out once you are having your implant treatment, or they may even be cutting costs in ways that you had really rather not know about *or care to experience!*

The reality is that to have this type of dental work done right it does require an investment. Why do so many people find it worth the extra cost? Aside from its longevity and hygienic effects, an implant can be undistinguishable from your natural, perfect tooth. An implant can last the rest of your life. Given the proper care and maintenance, implants can be a "one-time investment."

The materials, titanium and porcelain, are strong and durable; these can almost endure for a patient lifetime. Implants are set into the jawbone or down on it so that your living bone and tissue grow into and around it, forming an unbreakable anchor. Your new tooth (or teeth) is custom designed to match your teeth and face and to fit right in.

So, how do you find out what fees are involved? A private, complimentary consultation will help determine the range of fees for your rejuvenation. Note this: The fees we quote include not just the implants, but also the completed teeth, and in fact all of the in-between steps, too. A distinct advantage. Here we can work together to find the best solution for you based on what you want to achieve. Once a fee is set, that's the fee, end of story, no matter what kind of changes happen or surprises we encounter along the way. The only times this wasn't the case was an odd situation where a patient disappeared for several years in the middle of treatment and we had to start over from the beginning, and in another instance where a patient had some mental health issues and was physically harming the implants at home with hand tools!

What's more, you'll get a chance to receive a very detailed understanding of what is possible for you, meet our staff of professionals, and get a tour of our leading-edge facility.

Prevent Pain, Save Money

Dental implants <u>help prevent</u> the many costly and often painful dental problems that can arise later. Other potential health problems are also eliminated since one's <u>nutrition</u> is returned to normal by a diet of healthy foods.

Chapter 10
Appointments, Fees, Billing, and Insurance Must Be Easy for You!

In Fact, It Should be Painless.

Do we make these things easy for patients? Absolutely! We recognize the importance of being able to get appointments and having a flexible schedule.

We help you understand the fees, billing, and what insurance will and won't do for you so you can be comfortable financially, too.

We work to make fees affordable while helping maximize your insurance coverage.

If any of these administrative business items (appointments, fees, billing, or insurance) don't feel easy or understandable from day one when you visit a dentist, keep looking. These items must be just as "painless" as your treatment! After all, this is the 21st century!

Financing Made Easy

We offer a generous financing plan for qualified individuals to help with larger procedures. Often, your dental insurance can help pay a percentage of the total costs. Since the dental implanting procedures can be designed to take place in gradual steps over time (versus one day), your investment can also be spread out as long as payment is complete when work is finished.

Why Deal with Insurance Companies Yourself?

For complex situations, we guarantee that you will get the maximum amount possible from your particular dental insurance plan. We deal with thousands of plans and file your insurance forms for you, helping you win in dealing with insurance companies.

Dental insurance is nowhere near a pay-all service, but it's important to get help in paying for preventive maintenance dental care, as much coverage as your plan will allow. We help you get what should be coming to you.

Dental insurance no longer buys what it did 30-40 years ago when it became common. In fact, the annual maximum benefit levels haven't changed much in three decades. Routinely these maximums range from $1,000 to $2,000 per year.

To make matters worse, many companies now try to use fine print to avoid paying your benefits. Knowing that this is a headache and hassle for patients, we do our very best to maximize your policy's benefits.

My teeth were a mess. After interviewing many doctors and options, Dr. Holtan was the way to go.

They extracted all my teeth under IV sedation and when I woke up, I had teeth and was ready to chew (with restrictions). A few months, a couple of visits and in 5 months...I'm done. Bring on the steak, beef jerky, peanuts and don't forget corn (on the cob). I hardly notice they are even there.

Did I say that I even have molars? The last time I chewed in the back of my mouth was about 10 years ago. If I were any better looking, I would say look out Hollywood.

The Doc and his staff were professional, caring, and even interested in my well-being. It was well worth the time and money (which is about average with others) and unlike a sports car or new bike, my teeth will literally be with me forever because I can take them with me. 10 thumbs up.

– Scott B., Naples, FL

Chapter 11
The Horrible Hidden Costs of NOT Doing Treatment

The big thing is this: unhandled **dental problems get worse. If you think you are having trouble now, look ahead. Imagine what it could be** like to suffer even more, to be forced to endure more pain. For most patients, doing nothing is almost a certain guarantee that problems will worsen. The dental, social, and psychological pains only worsen.

• The Pain of *romance snuffed* out

• The Pain of teeth that don't look good

• The Pain of tender, sensitive, uncomfortable teeth

• The Pain of <u>lost ability to enjoy</u> your foods

• The Pain of worsened nutrition and health

• The Pain of **outright or potential of pain every time you bite down**

• The Pain of <u>lessened self-confidence</u>

- The Pain of depleted friendships

- The Pain of withdrawal from friends and family due to social embarrassment

- The Pain of losing the attention of that "certain someone" you want noticing you

- The Pain of losing the promotion that should have been yours

- The Pain of ever-increasing unsightly gaps among your teeth that worsen as you grow older

- The Pain of threatened health: up to 2-4 times the risk of heart attack and stroke, worsened diabetes, arthritis that won't get better

- The Pain of increasingly *depleted physical energy*

- The Pain of the loss of your zest for life

- For some people, the Pain means depression, *a black cloud hanging over your life that won't go away*

We hope that none of these befall you. But, the longer you wait, one (or many more) of these pains most certainly will come upon you.

So, the costs of not getting dental implant treatment is far, far worse and can be the ultimate cost – your life cut short by neglecting, ignoring, hoping it will go away, putting it off, and just not facing up to the very real, dark implications of not doing what you should.

Don't let those little voices inside your head cast doubt that stops you. Don't let those little voices make you feel too embarrassed to get treatment…to do something about it. Take charge and get the treatment you deserve.

Enhance Your Career…Make More Money

For many executives, salespeople, realtors, small business owners, and anyone who deals with the public…their mouth is how they make their money. It is their communication, appearance, and self-confidence that allows them to get their jobs done and help others. Could you even imagine an entertainer or media person with unattractive teeth? Absolutely not! Thus, their "look" is critical to their success!

Guess what…your looks are vital for your success, too…if you need to get others to do things, to persuade them or win them over in some way. And who doesn't?

Dental implants could just possibly be the best dollars you'll ever invest – making you more able to influence others to your way of thinking…winning that promotion…making more sales…putting a lot more money into your pocket.

A Case of Investing in Yourself

Take the case of Jean. Jean was a stay-at-home mom, a well-educated woman with multiple talents but who had now chosen to go back into the workforce.

She had a problem: her teeth. Somehow, she had never gotten around to them during all those years while her kids were growing up. Yes, she had regular check-ups but never did anything about them. Now she needed her mouth to look good to be able to get a job that paid her fairly well.

She finally did get a job offer but it was one beneath her real skills as a person. Her offer was for $22,000. She also knew the job she could get if she looked right…if she could smile with ease…easily and often…the job would probably be around twice as much – $48,000…a BIG difference.

It was going to cost many thousands to get her teeth fixed up. Jean had the money, but she was investing it, saving it for the "future." She decided not to get her teeth fixed…she got the $22,000 a year job. While she's received a cost of living adjustment, she's found that there is an unspoken stigma around how she looks, which she knows is holding her back from a bigger raise or even a promotion.

Brenda was like Jean: a stay-at-home mom, well educated, multitalented. Brenda had missing teeth and smile problems galore. Brenda had been looking for a job offer and also had an offer for $22,000. There had been another job open in the same company for $48,000 a year and she also knew she would be unlikely to get the higher-paying job due to the problems with her smile and confidence being held back by her dental problems.

Her treatment was going to be many thousands plus. Even more than Jean. But Brenda was bright. She had saved the money just like Jean. Brenda was a thinker...she reasoned that even if she had a 10% return on her money sitting in the bank she would still be better off investing in herself so that she would have faster and bigger pay raises and would soon be eligible to apply for a higher-paying job in the company once her foot was in the door. She made the investment in her smile and within a year her salary had been raised twice to $30,000. With her new level of confidence, she feels she has a reasonable shot at getting promoted into a soon to be open position that pays $55,000. Even her boss thinks she will be perfect in the much bigger position.

Plus, getting the dental work done also gave her a substantial tax deduction. Not to mention all the other benefits of a healthy mouth that looked good and felt good. Brenda got her treatment done. She got her job...the one she really wanted...and the pay she deserved. She's also on to the next step with being even happier in her career.

You're Never Too Old for a Healthy Mouth

Not unless you have one foot in the grave and you are on your deathbed! If you were in that situation, you wouldn't be reading this!

Why is it then you can't be too old for needed dental care? I believe a significant part of the answer lies with the aforementioned effects of having a healthy mouth on extending the length of your life and improving the quality of it.

Another reason to maintain your health is for those you love around you. Remember, you can pass along your infection to them as we discussed earlier.

Another recent study showed that most folks who wind up in nursing homes wear an upper denture, but by the time they arrive things have gotten so bad in their mouth that they can no longer wear their dentures. A very unfortunate thing is that the *last memories they leave* behind for their grandchildren is grandma or grandpa *without any teeth*. The good news is that with our new methods no one has to think about this happening to their grandchildren, especially considering how fast treatment can be now with being in and out of the office with teeth attached to one's dental implants on the very same day.

Yet another reason: when you have teeth that work, that look good and feel good, your relationship with the world around you and within yourself is significantly better.

We discussed the importance of your smile being a vital tool of communicating – relating and promoting yourself in your work.

Your smile increases the pleasure others have in dealing with you and subsequently enhances all your relationships with others.

Even another reason: As you get older, material items, things, and gadgets become less important.

What becomes more important is how you feel, your overall health, and maintaining relationships with those you love.

Having a healthy, properly functioning mouth affects every one of these desirable qualities.

It Does Take Time but Less Than You Imagine!

Implants do take some time. But ask yourself this question: If my dental health is more important to my longevity than stopping smoking – just how important is my dental health?

According to one source, those with good dental health live 6.6 years longer lives while those who stopped smoking increased their life by only 5.2 years. If you are married, it's important to remember that most men die before their wives. This weighs on many couples' minds. Why not do everything you can to have your mate and love of your life with you for as many years as possible?

If you look at this as a careful judge, your gavel comes down with a pounding affirmative – **it is worth the time even if you feel you don't have it.** Like everything else worth having, it does take some time, but with the newest advances like All-on-4 and The Sclar "One Day" Technique it's never taken less time.

Now with today's technology, treatment is easier, more convenient, and takes less time than ever before. As mentioned before, two of the newest methods in use at Dr. Holtan's practice quite literally have you walking into the office one day and on the very same day leaving with solid teeth that feel as good as or even better than your natural teeth. Make the time for yourself – you are worth it.

Need I point out to you that <u>your spouse, partner, children, or grandchildren are counting on you</u>. Even if you are very busy making a living to provide for your loved ones, what would happen if you had a serious health problem from not getting and maintaining a healthy mouth?

How much income do you lose then? How much income do you lose by not having an attractive smile? (It is a lot more than you think.)

Hello, Dr. Holtan, I hope you have a few moments!

You solved an obviously gigantic problem for me, you also made me understand a little more about modern medicine, and I am all the more grateful to you! It is impossible to predict the effect of living with "removable" teeth, until the fact hits you, especially in our youth oriented, perfect teeth society! I was pretty lucky in all respects throughout my life, but suddenly there was this secret immobilizing nightmare which grew to extreme proportions. And voila, you took it away!

Over and over again I had searched the world web for implant information with all its gory details. That did not frighten me. What scared me most was the possibility that, due to bone loss, it could not be done in my case. That's why I kept those awful few "witch teeth." So, the second you told me that I was indeed a "good subject," my troubles were gone! Now I had gained some distance from myself and could think about what you really do! And here it gets by necessity, a little philosophical!

As many new medical technologies (micro and macro) are allowing astonishing diagnosis, changes and repairs of our physical ailments and the possibilities of their applications boggle not only my mind, it is usually only their medical function which is publicly praised. Obviously, precise technology creates a perfect result (including my teeth). But and here is my non-professional opinion, for a technical object to be integrated and functioning in a living body (mine), scientific knowledge and practical know-how must be fused to another human capability or talent that cannot be learned. Technology works according to observable.

Predictable natural events, our natural laws, and it is repetitive. And although the "ingredients" of life obey the same laws, the event which makes them play this surprising show of life, does not. So far in my opinion, "explanations" of life are basically reports of that most complicated "chemical behavior" of the more complex but few ingredients in which life manifests itself. However, the crucial event of having been programmed or having programmed themselves with the plan of life, is not understood. Moreover, every resulting entity is unique.

This essential difference between nature and manmade things seems to render the integration of both as extremely difficult. And if the attempt is successful despite those hurdles, it must be due to talent that escapes exact description and which I call intuitive, creative spontaneity. Am I qualified to say this? I don't care! I am living proof that you have it! And thank you again!

Maybe you would like a simpler explanation better: you artistically bring people back to real life while many others adjust heads around teeth! I will not go into detail about the simultaneous, successfully applied psychological "treatment" by you and your staff. Thank them all!

Obviously, my daily routines alone will cause me to think of you often. My thoughts will always be happy! Should you and your family ever have time during one of your New York trips to visit your son, my husband and I would love to buy you dinner in Manhattan. I would enjoy that very much.

– Karin F., New York

Chapter 12
Competence You Can Count On

Comparatively, few dentists have taken the time, the extra courses, seminars, and hands-on training to be able to perform dental implants at this high level.

"Implantology," as this art and science is called, requires specialized procedures, instrumentation, and equipment.

During the process, you and **Dr. Holtan** may have many options. You can rest assured that they know the pros and cons of each and can make them clear to you as part of a personal and candid discussion with you.

For years, Dr. Holtan's patients have referred their friends for their expertise, friendly communication, and ability to get results.

Dr. Holtan is a graduate of the Marquette University School of Dentistry and received the 2010 Award for Excellence in Implant Dentistry. He became a Fellow at the American Academy of Implant Dentistry in 2017 and has been a member and prestigious Diplomate of the American Board of Oral Implantology/Implant Dentistry since 2016.

Dr. Holtan teaches techniques to other dentists to help them help their patients better.

He is a dentist who performs both the surgical placement and reconstructive phases of implants (placing the teeth themselves). Thus, you do not have to see two or more doctors in two or three different places to get your implant dentistry done. His experience helping patients with debilitating conditions via dental implant therapies is extensive.

Dr. Holtan's commitment to "doing it right" and the ability to "handle just about anything" has won him the admiration of patients and other doctors.

I must give this entire office, A five star!!! They all work hard to fit appointments into your schedule. They are always there to give you their undivided attention. Dr. Holtan is without any doubt, the best I have ever had in my lifetime. I travel a great distance for his special care. I recommend without reservation. You will be totally satisfied.

– Rose M., Jasper Georgia

Report: What Happens to Patients Who Have Implants

(Based on a study of 350 dental implant patients)

1. Knowing what you know now, <u>would you have the treatment again</u>?

   98% said yes

2. Was the treatment <u>worth the investment</u>?

   98% said yes

3. Was there a significant improvement in your ability to eat and chew?

   97% said yes

4. Was there a significant improvement in appearance?

   98% said yes

5. Was there a significant overall improvement?

   96% said yes

We Can Be More Than Just Your Implant Dentist

Our staff is ready to help you so that your total dental experience is the same we'd want for ourselves.

As full-service dental practices, Dr. Holtan, DDS can help you with all the routine services you would expect, along with the ones that you rarely see in most average and typical dental offices.

Among the routine services we offer are examinations, cleanings, check- ups, conservative laser gum treatment, tooth-colored lifelike fillings, advanced x-rays and computerized dental diagnostics, crowns, bridges, and specialized cosmetic dentures. For those who have been offered only a dental bridge or a partial denture solution, we promise to find an implant solution that will work for you – usually that solution can be had at a similar fee as any less than ideal solutions you may have been offered.

Among the not commonly seen services are:

➤ <u>Dental Implant Therapy – To replace missing teeth and rebuild smiles, performing all aspects of the treatment, surgery, and restoration.</u>

➤ <u>Virtually Unbreakable Implant Teeth</u> – Thanks to new types of porcelain and tooth design, in many situations, the teeth can be made to be nearly impervious to breaking and chipping!

> <u>Cosmetic Dentistry Services</u> – Smile make-over based on computer assisted Smile design to give you the look you've always wanted. See the "after" before we even start!

> <u>Rapid Whitening</u> to give you white, bright teeth in about an hour.

> <u>Extreme Power Whitening</u> If Hollywood white is your goal, then this is the technique for you.

> Super-Strong tooth-colored materials so teeth don't look gray or dark at the gum line…giving natural looking teeth.

> Full cosmetic consultation for challenging, difficult situations – restoring smiling and chewing to how they should be.

> Bad Breath Evaluation and Treatment

> Advanced Computerized diagnostics for jaw, joint problems, and physiologically based dental reconstructions.

> Advanced three-dimensional x-rays.

> <u>Advanced Laser Gum (Periodontal) Therapy</u> – Which includes using dental lasers, plastic surgery for your gums to make them look right, regenerative surgery using bone grafts

to rebuild missing bone, and specialized antibiotics to treat resistant gum disease. Old-fashioned gum surgery is a thing of the past.

➢ Specialized, Full Customized Cosmetic Dentures – Teeth that look stunning and natural. Photos of our patients with these teeth fool even dentists who attend teaching lectures.

➢ <u>In the mouth digital cameras</u> – so you can see what we see when we look into your mouth.

➢ <u>FDA Approved Migraine Headache Prevention</u> – that is 77% effective in reducing migraine headaches!

➢ Many patients say they really like the fact that they don't get sent all over town for their services.

Dear Dr. Holtan & Staff,

I want to thank you so much for what you have done for me. The teeth have changed my life tremendously. I now have a job and my manager says it is an awesome transformation for me. I realize now that having a job changes people's lives tremendously. My personality has changed tremendously.

– Holly.

P.S. My manager loves my new smile!

Chapter 13
Is a Smile an Investment That Makes Sense to You?

The question is this: Is it really worth it to you? Every individual must decide for himself or herself just how valuable and important a smile is that looks great but also is comfortable for chewing. So much so that you literally forget your teeth are there.

Here's a small hint: What if your pay or income went up 12.5-14.25%?

This isn't a number concocted out of thin air; it's based on a study that discovered the actual pay increase found by some researchers.

And it makes a lot of sense. If you had two qualified people walk into your office to apply for a job, one in average clothes with a noticeable tooth issue and the other dressed nicely with a great smile, you'd offer the job to the one dressed nicely with a great smile. You'd identify with that person more and believe he or she would be a good representation of your business. This is reality.

Calculate How Much Your Smile Is Worth

Here's a quick exercise to tell you how much a smile may be worth for you. Go ahead and multiple your salary by the additional percentage of pay or income; be conservative and use the 12.5%.

Here's a chart to help you, just in case you don't have a calculator nearby.

YEARS UNTIL RETIREMENT

Income 5 years	12.5% 10 years	14.25% 20 years
$30,000 $18,750	$3750 $37,500	$4350 $ 75,000
$35,000 $21,875	$4375 $43,750	$4988 $ 87,500
$40,000 $25,000	$5000 $50,000	$5700 $100,000
$45,000 $28,125	$5625 $56,250	$6413 $112,500
$50,000 $31,250	$6250 $62,500	$7125 $125,000
$55,000 $34,375	$6875 $68,750	$7838 $137,500

$60,000	$7500	$8550
$37,500	$75,000	$150,000
$65,000	$8125	$9263
$40,625	$81,250	$162,500
$70,000	$8750	$9975
$43,750	$87,500	$175,000
$75,000	$9375	$10,688
$46,875	$93,750	$187,500

Now multiply that additional amount of pay times the number of years you plan to continue working. For someone who makes $30,000 a year who plans to retire in 20 years, the additional pay just for having a nice smile for those 20 years could be worth at least $75,000 in today's dollars.

When piled on top of all the other enormous benefits: increased confidence; greater self-esteem; enhanced personal and business relationships; being treated better by those around you; easily making more friends and business contacts; having an increased ability to influence your associates, co-workers or colleagues, customers, friends and even the next door neighbor; clients; the scale tips overwhelmingly (bang!) to the side of having a great smile.

Now don't you agree that this investment pays dividends every day of your life? For many people it really isn't an option; it is truly a necessity.

All I get is compliments on my new teeth! My friends want to know if I used a whitening system to get them to look this good. They never even guess that they are dentures. Dr. Holtan, you and your staff deserve all the credit. You were patient and kind and did the most wonderful job. I can't thank you enough.

– Dottie D., Cleveland, OH

Chapter 14
People Always Look at Your Teeth… What Do They See?

It's scientifically proven that people see your smile or teeth as the **first or second thing they notice when they look at you!** Did you realize this? In some studies, the researchers report the first thing seen is the eyes, and in other studies the answer is <u>the smile</u>.

Either way, when you come into contact with other people, they ARE going to notice your teeth and smile no matter what since the main ways we communicate with other people are with our mouths and eyes.

Even animals observe the mouths of other animals and whether or not the animal they are meeting is showing teeth or not.

People are drawn to beautiful things by instinct. Studies with babies prove that they are drawn to people who are more beautiful, based on the placement of the eyes, nose, and mouth on the face and the symmetry of those features. Beauty on the face can be either enhanced with a smile or negated instantly when the person smiles. A beautiful smile plays a huge importance in how attractive other people see you. The proportions that go into a great smile, even smiles created on the same day, is something that demands great attention to detail and something we pride ourselves on looking at carefully with each patient.

You probably already knew this just by using common sense. And now after 20-30 years, your common sense has been verified by scientific evidence overwhelmingly proving the importance of a great smile and how you are perceived and treated by others in every situation in life.

For a better understanding of this, we will discuss *8 different ways that a nice smile can influence your daily walk in life.*

The #1 Way a Nice Smile Influences Your Daily Walk of Life and Treats You in All Situations

What has science proven? The bottom line is this: the better you look, <u>the better you are treated by others</u>. It cannot be emphasized enough that being more attractive has distinct advantages.

Generally, people greatly underestimate this reality. Like it or not, people who are seen by others as attractive are thought to be smarter, better at their jobs, more talented, more kind, and even more honest!

This is true throughout our entire society at every level from the working class to those with great wealth. Your smile and teeth play a large part in how much other people want to be around you and how much they like and believe you.

Just by having a great smile you become more likely to be promoted in your job... more attractive and likely to find your best mate in life...more likely to be wanted by others in friendships...and even more likely to be trusted.

We'll cover the remaining seven ways in the next chapters.

Chapter 15
Three More Ways a Great Smile Can Influence Your Day

The #2 Way a Nice Smile Influences Your Daily Walk of Life

Social Advantages of Looking Good and Having a Great Smile

People that are good-looking enjoy social advantages without even trying. They are seen as smarter and liked better. They are seen as more desirable and as people with better personalities.

Nice-looking people have a better ability to persuade those around them and are far more likely to receive help from others. Behavioral science (how people react in situations and in relation to others) continues to support this.

Imagine how quickly you'll run to the mirror to see what your new smile will look like after your dental work is finished on the same day. Imagine how much you'll actually like appearing in family photos again...have you avoided them in the past? If so, it's time to change this. You are an important part of your family and their legacy and need to be counted.

#3 Way a Nice Smile Influences Your Daily Walk of Life

Attractive School Children Get into Less Trouble in School and Are Seen as Being Smarter

A landmark study by Dion in 1972 showed that attractive school children were viewed as less naughty when misbehaving compared to children who were less attractive.

Twenty years later, in 1992, a study by Ritts, Patterson, and Tabbs found that teachers perceive that attractive students are more intelligent than less unattractive students.

If you're a student, your teeth can make or break you! This type of teacher bias is far from fair – but it's the way things are. Are you or your children ostracized because of teeth issues? Think about this...but also think of the flip side of it. What if you were a teacher with a missing tooth? How would the students perceive you?

The #4 Way a Nice Smile Influences Your Daily Walk of Life

Good-Looking Political Candidates

Are More Likely to Win Elections!

Few people would admit to voting for a candidate because they were more attractive. A Canadian study proved this bias (Efran and Patterson in 1976).

Political candidates who were attractive got 2 ½ times the number of votes of unattractive candidates. Voters of course denied that their votes were influenced by whether a candidate was good looking or not…but yet it is true.

While it's unlikely that you will have an interest to be elected to a public office, people around you will be "casting votes" for or against you either intentionally or sublimely based on many factors including your smile. You can choose to influence those perceptions with our help and with the new technologies being discussed in this book.

We'll review the final four ways a nice smile influences your daily walk of life next.

Chapter 16
Four More Ways a Great Smile
Influences Your Life

The #5 Way a Nice Smile Influences Your Daily Walk of Life

Being Attractive Makes Getting Jobs Easier

A 1990 study (Mack and Rainey) showed that being nice looking and well-groomed accounted **more in the hiring decision than job qualifications**!

The #6 Way a Nice Smile Influences Your Daily Walk of Life

Attractiveness Influences the Law and Justice System

A study in Pennsylvania in 1980 by Steward showed that good-looking people received more favorable treatment in the justice system. If you have to attend civil court for any reason, even when appealing a parking ticket, this could play a role in the ultimate outcome.

Of course, this would also apply to the attorneys who represent their clients throughout the justice system. Having or getting an attractive, head-turning smile is something some attorneys have quietly told us is one of their secrets beyond simply being competent and genuinely interested in helping their clients.

Finally, strangely but not really surprisingly, after understanding all of the studies pointing to smiles, attractiveness, and other people's perceptions, one study also found that attractive people were far more likely to avoid jail time in criminal situations. If they did receive a jail sentence, it was much lighter.

The #7 Way a Nice Smile Influences Your Daily Walk of Life

You Can Make More Money if You Have a Great Smile

Attractive workers get paid ***on average up to 14% more*** than unattractive workers.

This was shown to be true in both the U.S. and Canada (Hammermesh and Biddle, 1994).

The #8 Way a Nice Smile Influences Your Daily Walk of Life

Men and Women Agree That Attractive Teeth Are Better

Both sexes respond to attractiveness in similar ways. Having a better smile makes you better in all kinds of ways to both men and women.

Some of our patients report having more fun dating and even a renewed romantic life after getting their smile back or by having it improved.

Dear Melissa,

About 2 years ago I was faced with very serious dental problems and needed multiple dental implants. I consulted with several implant specialists and dentists in the Naples area and was charged considerable consultation fees in the process. About 16 months ago I contacted your office and Dr. Holtan evaluated my situation and came up with a very effective treatment plan – all without charge, I might add.

Dr. Holtan did the extensive work with utmost professionalism. The implants have been in place for over a year now. My quality of life

143

has improved tremendously because of his excellent work and I am very grateful to him and his staff. I gladly recommend him to anyone in need of detailed implant work."

– Irma W., Naples FL

Chapter 17
Not Having a Good-Looking Smile Used to Be Optional – Not Anymore

While a good-looking smile may have been an option before, that's not the case today. You may or may not know the exact advantages for you of having a great smile. Stop and think about it for a moment. What about your job? Your relationships with others? Your ability to make friends? Your climb up the career ladder?

Do you think you'd be more confident in yourself knowing you have a great smile?

You Can Even Help Someone You Care About – Here's How

Think about those around you whom you care about the most…your loved ones, friends, and family.

Could their attractiveness and likeability be changed for the better with improvements in their smile? You could be doing them a huge favor by influencing them to get a great smile!

You see it almost every day. People buy all kinds of expensive clothing just to look and feel better. Many women spend thousands of dollars a year on hair treatments, nail jobs, and expensive makeup to look the best they can. And this goes on…year after year…at untold sums of money.

Now there is nothing wrong with this, because those things have an influence on how one feels and impacts relationships and work as well. However, now that you know the importance and effect of a beautiful smile, do you think that a portion of this time, money, and effort could be better spent by improving a smile for decades of use?

These temporary beauty enhancements would be greatly improved if the smile was at the same level. How many people have you seen with the most fashionable clothes, but have dark, stained, broken-down, or just ugly teeth that ruin their appearance? Sadly enough, you see far too many!

The best news is that a new smile lasts far longer than any of those temporary enhancements. We've intentionally selected new cosmetic materials for dental implants that are made to last a lifetime. One particular type of dental porcelain we now use is *virtually unbreakable*; meaning that the biting surface of the teeth cannot wear out with everyday chewing! Yes, you could say, it is a never-ending goal of ours to want dentistry (and smiles) to last a very long time.

If this same kind of information about unbreakable teeth isn't being presented to you either in person by another doctor or in materials you've received from any other practice, be aware that the materials you would likely receive with treatment are likely to be of an earlier generation and because of such are prone to chipping and breakage. Once again, now that you know the differences, you are armed with information to either ask "why" or simply to seek out another opinion.

There's another aspect about this topic that you may not have considered: If you have teeth that are in need of restoration, your physical health can be affected, too. You won't be eating salads, fruits, and vegetables when your teeth aren't right.

Studies show that salads, fruits, and vegetables are clearly linked to preventing dozens of different diseases, most of them degenerative diseases such as heart disease, cancer, diabetes, and high blood pressure.

You'll read a lot more about the connection between eating and your health later.

Chapter 18
Shocking News –
All Dentists Don't Use the
Latest Techniques.

Some in fact are still using technologies from the 20th and even 19th centuries.

Choosing a dentist for dental implants or any type of dental work can be a difficult task. That's because you know that choosing the right one can make life so much easier! No one wants to make a mistake!

Dentistry has progressed to the point where a dental implant can be inserted in one hour while you are in the dentist chair over lunch. A tooth can be rebuilt in one dental appointment. A tooth-colored (invisible) crown, in fact several, can be made in roughly an hour.

Teeth can look yellow going into the dentist's office but be brighter than snow coming out – and that changes your entire life because now you are flashing a big smile to everyone you meet! You're acting in alignment with how you feel about yourself and it shows to other people. There's something about a big, beautiful smile that brings out the best in every one of us.

Not All Dentists Are the Same!

But there's something you should always consider and be aware of: dentists are not all the same. The initials may all look alike but the men and women behind the initials are anything but standardized.

Dentists vary in their skill sets and educational background as well as experience. All dentists go to dental school and start out with the same amount of education and skills; however, what they do in the next 10 to 20 years becomes the foundation for their entire career and the basis of who they can serve best. 95% of the profession does the basics very well but _**only 5% go on to be at the top**_ *of the food chain in knowledge, skills, and judgment*.

Some dentists are blessed with experiences where they work with dozens of people who need an implant, while others receive referrals of dozens of patients who need complex dentistry on their natural teeth. During the time these dentists spend with these patients, they are accumulating vast knowledge on how to work with all the variations that arise during implant or reconstructive dentistry.

All this knowledge is to your benefit. If you walk into our offices for these types of services you are capitalizing on all that kind of experience, which is the best teacher in life.

Your Childhood Dentist Is an Example

Another way to explain why all dentists are not the same is to look at the dentist you had as a child. A dentist who serves the pediatric (child) population has excellent skills in allaying fears about dentistry. He is very patient and may also have children of his own. He is great at identifying potential problems with permanent adult teeth and wisdom teeth that are on their way but not fully developed, and an expert at using braces to straighten teeth as well as using sealants to protect the teeth from decay.

However, children rarely need implants, cosmetic crowns of any kind, or even cosmetic teeth whitening. In fact, pediatric dentists are the first to tell you that children must wait until they are 18 years old before you consider an implant or teeth whitening for them. The knowledge and information your childhood dentist had was limited to just these things.

While childhood dentists are experts at child problems, implant dentists are dentists that are experts at solutions for replacing missing teeth. Some implant dentists are also experts at rebuilding, reconstructing, and saving what can be saved with one's natural teeth – something the profession calls reconstructive dentistry.

While the child dentist works for years to perfect techniques that help children, the implant or reconstructive dentist has been working for years to perfect how to insert implants in newer, faster ways so there is no embarrassment about missing teeth. The reconstructive dentist will also have been perfecting how to combine life-like cosmetic crowns with safe teeth-whitening procedures, so people don't experience the shame of not having as bright of a smile as everyone else. These perfectionists are often out there giving seminars to fellow dentists and leading and teaching others how to perfect their skills. These types of perfectionists fall into the Expert Dentist Type 3 Category, which we will discuss in a bit.

Not All Dentists Provide Celebrity Smiles

Similarly, the dentist your parents chose for you as a child or teenager would not be the right dentist for you if you needed your smile to look like that of a celebrity, to have pearly whites that are absolutely stunning, or even if you simply wanted to get back a smile that shows that all the teeth you have are sound and healthy in your mouth.

Working with celebrity teeth is probably one of the most exacting and precise types of dentistry a dentist can do. Celebrities are on a pedestal and the public looks for every little flaw they may have. If there is one tooth that is even a little bit abnormal, let alone darker or more yellow in color than the other teeth, that celebrity will be poked at by the public. Heaven forbid the time when a celebrity is in the public and missing a tooth! The media would have a heyday with that!

Thus, the dentist focusing on cosmetics and "celebrity teeth" is a perfectionist in every form. The dentist your parents sent you to may never have had to be a perfectionist at this level. He or she would have focused on being reasonably good at everyday procedures instead of these areas requiring more education and expertise. See the difference? Your choice of dentists matters a lot.

Dentists May Specialize in Traumatic, Serious Cases

If you have had a traumatic accident that has affected your teeth and left you with missing teeth as well as other problems, you will need and want a dentist who has the most technological advancements along with the most knowledge and experience.

For example, here's one type of case where an ordinary dentist would never do. Mary was in a serious car accident and ended up with facial injuries that were quite severe. She ended up losing some teeth in the process, as well as suffering damage to her jaw, lips, and palate. She needed full mouth dental reconstruction and also an oral and plastic surgery reconstruction because of the damage to her tissues.

The dentist she found had advanced degrees in dentistry, internships that provided the foundational experience needed to understand these cases and how to set up their treatment plans, and advanced training in implants, cosmetic dentistry, and bridgework, too. The dentist brought in a specialized oral surgeon for her situation to handle the reconstruction of her facial tissue.

Although Mary's recovery took a long time because of the type of injuries, her dentist team carefully reconstructed her mouth, teeth, and jaw so she could eat, talk, and move her lips as before. Without the right dentist in charge, Mary may have had eating disabilities for the rest of her life.

In Mary's case, a dentist starting a new practice would never have been the best choice because of the whole mouth restoration. Her childhood dentist also would not have been a good choice, even though she might have felt the most comfortable with him. A cosmetic dentist would not have been a good match either since this involved far more than dentistry on natural teeth. Lastly, her basic, average adult dentist would have also been out of his or her league because of the complexities. Once again, based on the situation, a special level of expert (Type 3 Dentist) was required.

Consider Your State of Oral Health Right Now

If you have been troubled with gum disease for as long as you can remember, it's possible you may have to take another look at the dental care you have been receiving.

Is it possible that the method used to treat you in your current dental office is not the most advanced? Is the method used to treat you one that was good for a while, but now needs to be updated?

One sure, easy to spot, sign that the practice is behind the times is if the dental hygienist is just "scraping" your teeth with old-fashioned metal instruments without the use of another more high-tech instrument called the ultrasonic cleaner (yes, even for a basic cleaning!). The ultrasonic cleaner removes not only tartar, but it breaks up the "homes" that bacteria make along your gum line. As it cleans it also applies a disinfectant around the gums where the bacteria hide, which further prevents them from creating infectious problems. Regular hand instruments, besides removing tartar, do none of these things. If that wasn't enough, those old-fashioned instruments hurt far more than the modern ultra-sonic cleaner!

There are also new ways of literally zapping the bacteria in the gum pockets with laser energy to eliminate them before they have another chance to reproduce. Yet, if a dentist or hygienist hasn't kept up with the advancements in this aspect of dentistry, you certainly won't find this technology or protocol in that practice AND you will be lucky if any gum condition you have stays stable for even 10 years.

The science now shows that traditional gum disease treatment, while slowing progression, never truly halts deterioration. It is only by the use of newer methods like bacteria DNA testing for the correct antibiotic to use for an individual patient's specific bacteria along with laser gum therapy can this disease be stabilized fully and even halted. If "traditional" is all you've been offered, then perhaps it's time to move to another practice in command of where the science stands!

Why worry about this? Well, the problem is that when gum disease progresses as it does when it is treated via outdated traditional methods, over the course of 10 years you could easily lose more teeth than necessary. This tooth loss then causes a whole host of new problems (such as eating less nutritious foods, premature facial aging, the need for more dental work, etc.) and of course makes you even more at risk for continued tooth loss. It's a repetitive cycle! Also remember from our earlier discussions, even heart disease is linked to gum disease infections especially when the gums are in a state of chronic inflammation.

You might even be shying away from getting a tooth replaced because of the cost of conventional dental implants and the down time, but the fact is that there are NEW ways to get dental implants that are more economical than the old versions and that will save you time as compared to even five years ago.

Chapter 19
Six Considerations to Make When Choosing a Dentist

Another major purpose of this patient guidebook is to give you the information and tools you need to choose a dentist that's right for you. No dentist can claim to have the skills to help every single patient, and we don't make that claim either! We want you to know how to choose a dentist so you can find the dentist who exactly matches your needs regardless of where you might live and be reading this.

Through our years of experience and thousands of hours of post-doctoral training, we at Dr. Holtan's office in Southwest Florida have uncovered the most common mistakes to avoid when choosing a dentist.

We know you'll be amazed at a few of them and will say to yourself, "I'm so glad I had the chance to read the guidebook before I went looking for a dentist!" With a few more of the common mistakes, you will most likely think to yourself, "Well, that makes a lot of sense!" And with a few of them, you will most likely say, "I knew that and I'm glad I'm not the only one!"

When you decide to choose a dentist, if you use this guidebook as your reference, you'll find that it will help you form the basis of a strong, informed, and wise decision on who your dentist should be and who is the right dentist for you.

In the coming section, we'll cover the following recommendations about what's critical about any dental practice or dentist you might consider.

➤ Consideration #1 – Make sure the initial visit is free.

Otherwise, you could end up with a bill you never wanted and shouldn't have had to pay. And really, why should anyone pay to see if a dentist is a good match for you? We'll get into more of the reasoning on this shortly.

➤ Consideration #2 – Make sure your dentist has a proven track record.

Otherwise, you could end up with archaic methods and procedures that cause more pain than what you should have to endure or procedures that are not long-lasting in their effects.

> **Consideration #3 – Work with as few dentists as possible.**

Otherwise, you could end up in the middle of a battle of wills between dental professionals and feel as if you are tossed back and forth with no continuity. You will also likely find that one staff you get along with and the other one you dread seeing at very visit. Never a good situation when one is considering more complex types of dentistry!

> **Consideration #4 – Find a dentist who makes office business procedures easy – in fact, makes them painless!**

Otherwise, you could end up wasting far too much time dealing with insurance companies and their billing staff, wasting time with double-booked appointments, and tearing your hair out with billing errors and have to prove that you are right.

> **Consideration #5 – Find a dentist who thinks carefully about long-term smile health and long-term oral health. If you ask the dentist to explain "lifetime risk" and he or she can't do so, or hasn't heard of this concept, this is not a practice you belong in!**

Otherwise, there's a good chance you'll end up with more dental work than what is necessary.

> **Consideration #6 – Find a dentist within a reasonable travel distance. Be aware of the risks of "Vacation Dentistry."**

Otherwise, you could end up spending thousands more dollars on dental emergencies and have difficulties getting the original dentist to help if there are problems.

You Need a Dentist Who Is Savvy About Dental Advancements

Everyone is at times a bit overwhelmed in this age of technical information. Technology is a good thing because it means that everyday citizens get to benefit from the latest advancements that even the wealthiest of 50 years ago could not have imagined.

You rely on your licensed professionals (accountants, physicians, and dentists) to apply the very best technology that matters the most for you and to make it as uncomplicated to us a layperson as possible.

The problem is in thinking or in having a mindset that all dentists are actually USING the latest and most important advancements. We've been touching on this throughout the guidebook. By now, you know that all dentists are not keeping on top of the most important advancements.

In fact, very few dentists are on the leading edge of the most current details needed to keep you from losing teeth or to give you back parts of your dental health that you may be missing, and to do all of this in the fastest time possible and in a virtually painless manner.

You Need a Dentist Who Can Make Complex Dentistry Simple to Understand

Additionally, even in cases where the dentist has been keeping up, these advancements aren't always discussed with you, the patient, in terms you can understand. This leads to confusion. Anytime we as humans are confused, we are less likely to make sound judgments – even when it comes to our health! We hear this from patients coming to discuss their dental problems, and because of this we have a "no confusion" promise in that we'll do whatever it takes to make whatever dentistry we might recommend simple for you to understand.

Our dental offices were created so you can experience friendly, gentle dentistry that produces proven results – a great smile and healthy teeth for life and to not be confused by any choices being offered. We have a "no confusion" rule. Nothing proceeds or happens if there is an ounce of confusion!

If you are someone who wants teeth that look good and feel good, and if what most of what we've been discussing in this guidebook appeals to you, you'll like the practices of Dr. Holtan. Even with that being the case, you still have to determine if our office and our services have exactly what you need.

You'll be able to make many preliminary decisions from reading this patient guidebook. Then you'll want to take the rest of your questions directly to Dr. Holtan. You can be assured of an honest evaluation and assessment.

Read on and you'll discover common mistakes to avoid when choosing a dentist. Get ready to expand your mind and intelligence! This information may not be found anywhere else, all in one place, and specifically written in an easy-to-understand manner with you, as an individual patient, in mind.

Dear Dr. Holtan,

I am so pleased with my recent implant that my only regret is that I didn't find out about such remedies much sooner. It's difficult to describe the "difference," the implant feels like a part of me, nothing gets under it and it isn't taken out to be cleaned. It just couldn't be more real except of course; it will never ache! Thanks again!

– Charlotte R., Fort Myers, FL

Chapter 20

Consideration #1 When Selecting a Dentist

Make Sure the Initial Visit Is Free

You Shouldn't Have to Pay for the First Meet and Greet Visit

The first thing that can go wrong – if you don't watch out – occurs if you believe that an initial visit, especially a "meet and greet" or talking visit, isn't free.

Here's an example of how a scenario can play out. Peter is a very busy business owner. He's an entrepreneur and like most people who own their own businesses has to budget his time carefully between all the demands.

He's so busy working all the time that his wife has to make all his appointments for him. She made an appointment with Dr. Jones, a local dentist whom a neighbor had recommended. Peter thought he was going to go to his visit to simply talk a bit about his dental concerns. However, immediately after being seated by Dr. Jones' assistant, he found himself having a full set of x-rays being taken, and then, instead of a personal discussion before looking at his teeth, Dr. Jones simply said "open wide," picked around a bit, barely spoke to him, tapped some things into his computer with his back turned, and then scurried off to the next room without even a short "goodbye" or "nice to meet you."

Peter knew he had a few dental problems but what he didn't know, and was deciding, was whether he even wanted to see Dr. Jones as his dentist! There was no rapport but there was a bill for services that Peter didn't really want that day.

To make matters worse, the solutions the front office assistant printed out for him were simply a bunch of medical codes and completely confusing. His confusion led to him doing nothing for another year until ultimately one of the teeth he had been concerned about became extremely painful and required an expensive, and what could have been unnecessary, emergency root canal visit.

Your First Visit Is Similar to a Date in Some Ways

Now there are many things here that actually went wrong, but the bottom line is that at the initial visit, it should be considered like a date. You're meeting the dentist to see if there's a match, as two people would meet each other at a coffee shop to see if there's anything further to pursue.

You never want to jump into some program of dental treatments, especially at the first visit.

A first visit is an investment of the dentist's time as well as it is an investment of your time. There should be no charge for this.

Would you think of paying someone for their time if it didn't work out? No! Never, as it is a mutual investment of time. Sometimes they work out and other times they don't. If your dentist doesn't work out on your first visit, there are plenty of others you can find to try.

Dentists often guarantee your first visit as one that is free. However, some don't and proceed full speed ahead to expect that you are already their patient. But you aren't – yet.

Then You Have to Enforce Your Beliefs!

It takes a very strong-willed person who sees the inappropriateness of this type of behavior to walk out and never come back.

And since most people like to carefully select their battles in life, this might not be chosen as one of yours. You might end up feeling like you're stuck with a particular dental practice that you'd rather not be a member of.

You have a right to check out a new dentist. By no means are you tied to this first dentist after a simple consultation.

If There's No Evidence of These Two Things at the First Visit, Move on to Another Dental Practice

At that first appointment, you're looking for:

• **Rapport between the two of you.**

Is the rapport like that of a new friend that you can already tell cares for you?

Does the dentist and his team really listen to you?

Were their office forms standard and cold or did they use a caring application that asked questions about how your dental situation had been impacting your life?

Were they really trying to find out how to help you on your need versus their pre-conceived notions about you?

• **Common Sense in what the dentist thinks you need to have done.**

What do you think you need to have done? What does the dentist say you need to have done?

Are the answers similar, and if not does their reasoning seem sound?

Did the dentist ask about both how your problems are affecting you and what kind of answer you are looking for that you would be happy with?

If the reasoning doesn't make sense to you or there's no effort to really match solutions to what would make you happy when you are finished with any dentistry, you'll either want to move on to the next doctor. If you do go through with getting a treatment plan or options, take those recommendations and get a second opinion at a Type 3 Expert level dentist.

Sometimes what we don't know about our teeth is due to lack of knowledge. This is understandable as you aren't a dentist. But sometimes the dentist has plans for you that really don't fit your situation.

Here's an example. Lou was a television show host and had a job where he was in the public's eye quite a bit. He never knew ahead of time that a public appearance was scheduled and had to be ready always, just in case.

Lou visited a dentist for the first visit who, with little to no discussion or reasoning, told him he needed braces and that his teeth should be reconstructed to look more masculine. There was also a bill waiting for Lou at the end of the visit. On the bill, the dental office wrote "consultation for braces."

And then the dentist was ready to schedule the next appointment for the braces!

"Whoa, Mr. Dentist! All I came in for was a consultation! No one in the show biz world ever said my teeth looked feminine, and I like them the way they are. The only place where they are crowded is in the lower bottom row where no one even views them – and all that means is more cleaning on your hygienist's part!"

Clearly, there was no match between this dentist and the patient. Lou did what you would want to do too and that was keep looking!

Get a Guarantee from Your Dentist

The moral of this chapter is to **make sure your first visit to the new dentist is guaranteed free. Without this guarantee, you may be walking into a surprise you would rather avoid. At Dr. Holtan's our initial "meet and great" and "talking visits" are** *always* **free to you.**

What You Really Want at Any Dental Office

At the practice of Dr. Holtan in South Florida, you'll notice a difference the moment you step into our state-of-the-art facility, designed for your comfort.

Honestly, though, a far more important aspect of our unique dental practices is our staff. They are people's people who enjoy giving great service and they really listen to you.

No Scolding and No Embarrassment – Guaranteed

Many of our patients have remarked to us what a friendly, upbeat office we have. We take personal pride in being an office that our patients like to come to.

If you haven't been to a dentist in a long while, you can be assured of not being embarrassed or scolded.

Listen, we know it can be hard to come in even though you know you need to do so. We won't make it any harder. We work to make it easy, so you can feel relieved about that!

We work with you individually to help you get the right kind of dental care that looks good, feels good, and helps keep your teeth for a lifetime.

You'll benefit from the latest technology available in equipment, materials, and technology so you not only have great dental health, but you also have a great smile. You'll enjoy a friendly, upbeat atmosphere of open communication.

We answer your questions, and work to understand your concerns.

We also offer something that is very unusual in a dental office…

"Can't Go Wrong" First Complete Dental Physical Examination – GUARANTEED or It's FREE

While many offices might be willing to guarantee a short "meet and greet" visit to be free to you, almost no one will place a similar guarantee on a physical examination appointment.

To make it easier for you to choose, we've also created a special guarantee that goes beyond what others might be doing. It's simply this: If after the first clinical examination you decide we aren't right for each other, you can leave and pay nothing.

Why would we do this? Because in 96 cases out of 100, our patients choose to stay. They like who we are and what we do for them – and we think you will, too.

Chapter 21

Consideration #2 When Selecting a Dentist

Make Sure Your Dentist Has a Proven Track Record

A dentist with a proven track record of advanced education, teaching, and the endorsements of practicing colleagues of his services to you goes a long way. Ask for all of these things!

Three Types of People & Three Types of Dentists

Have you ever noticed there are three types of people found in every corner of life?

These three types are:

• Type 1 – Those who don't go the distance to meet a goal

- Type 2 – Those that do meet a goal and are then satisfied with it and become lazy about new goals

- Type 3 – Those who meet a goal and are so passionate about it that they can't help themselves to go far beyond it and keep growing and goal setting year after year after year

These three types of people behavior apply to the dental profession as well.

Thankfully, there are almost no examples of a **Type #1 Dentist** – someone attempting to practice dentistry without a license. Our government has determined that if one doesn't attend dental school and meet certain basic abilities and standards that one can't simply say "I'm a dentist" and start treating people!

The Type #2 Dentist (The Average Dentist)

Very Common, but Very Likely Not for Those with Major Dental Problems

The second type, the Type #2 Dentist, **comprises 95%** of the dental profession. This is someone who went to school to get their basic dental knowledge on how to deal with average problems in average patients. Most patients need dentists just like this. That is a very good thing since the majority of the dental profession is composed of Type #2 Dentists.

Another common trait of the Type #2 "average" Dentist is in how much (or little) he continues to invest in higher learning. Once he's out of dental school, he seldom wants to invest in the latest technology that allows the most pain-free method to clean teeth or fix your teeth or to place an implant. Yes, average people with average programs are okay with an "average" dentist, but what if you have complex problems?

It's not unusual that upon achieving the license to become a dentist that he said to himself, "I'm done with all that schooling! I know everything I need to know now, and I'll do just the bare minimum to keep my license active." He often looks for the cheapest ways to meet the minimal educational requirements to maintain his license. Oftentimes it's via magazine articles with a quiz on the subject matter. There's no debate in the profession that this kind of education, while technically fulfilling educational requirements, pales in comparison to symposiums complete with live lectures, back and forth discussions between the professors and the doctors at the lecture, small discussion groups focusing on specific patient situations and ways to solve them, and in some cases even treating patients during the course. Which type of educational routine would you prefer your dentist to be a part of? High-level learning or back of a magazine learning?

Although it is true that a Type #2 Dentist will know the basic information, it's important to realize that dentistry is a field that involves an awful lot of topics, many of which require a much greater understanding beyond the basics. This includes things such as:

• dental implants

• cosmetic dentistry

• teeth whitening

• cosmetic fillings and crowns

• cavities

• safe amalgam removal

• tooth sealants

• gum disease detection and treatment

• digital x-rays

• dental lasers

• special protocols to eliminate pain with injections and treatment

• and a lot more

Literally, it's impossible to be a real expert in any given area when one only graduates with a basic dental school degree and especially when "just the minimum" to maintain the doctor's license has been his educational goal since graduating.

The Bottom Line Is Your Mouth Is Different

But – and this is a big BUT – every mouth is different. Every mouth needs custom attention in some way so that the patient gets the best results. And that customization comes from three things:

- Additional seminars and training – in fact, hundreds and even thousands of hours to achieve mastery

- Additional successful results on patients

- Gathering together similar experts and sharing high-level knowledge far beyond the basics

The Type #3 Dentist – The Expert Level Dentist

Thus, the third type of professional in the dental field – and as any other field – is the one whom everyone admires because he can't stop learning. He HAS TO go get additional training. It's a drive in him to be the best he can be. Approximately **5% of the profession is in this category**!

Maybe he does this through seminars that offer board designations, or maybe he even goes back to school for an advanced dental degree.

While obtaining this additional training, the professors are discussing all the small details that can affect that type of dental procedure. Some of the details of your case may be included in that training.

Then when discussions arise about the procedure, this type of dentist listens intently and learns the nuances of each situation and condition. He is equipping himself with hundreds of scenarios where each may be a little bit different when a procedure is performed. This is how he becomes a true expert.

This is the type of dentist that you want working on your teeth, especially if you have complex dental problems. One that can't help himself but be driven by an insatiable curiosity to learn everything that is to be learned about dentistry and special classes of procedures that solve patients' most difficult problems. One that masters a procedure and is not satisfied – he has to master another and another.

The Type #3 Dentist – The Expert Dentist – Is One You Can Have Confidence In

Where do you fit into this picture? Think about your situation a bit. Does it need "average" or truly "expert?" If your answer was "expert," then when you are examined in the dental chair of this type of dentist, you can have confidence in the results that will be received.

Good dentistry comes as a result of the combination of education... ongoing professional post-doctoral training and teaching...talent... experience...and the commitment to doing it right.

You'll discover that Dr. Holtan has a passionate commitment to give you quality dentistry that looks good and feels good and you'll experience what it means to be seen by the Type #3 Dentist.

If you have a challenging dental situation, you'll like what Dr. Holtan and his staff can do for you.

Why? Because you can expect they will employ all of their wide-ranging diagnostic and treatment methods to figure out what works best for your situation. You can also see before and after pictures of patients who were told or believe that they had "hopeless" situations when in fact, thanks to their finding Type #3 Dentists, there was actually a lot of hope at **www.NoMoreDentures.net.**

By the way, Dr. Holtan has ongoing Free Public Seminars on the latest dental technology and how it can give you a beautiful smile.

Thank you Dr. Holtan!

I want to express how pleased I am with the result of your full mouth reconstruction. Thanks to you and your professional staff, implant dentistry has given me a healthier, stronger, and more aesthetically pleasing appearance. The process was painless and exceedingly efficient (just six visits). Thank you for all your fine work.

– Kevin G., Naples, FL

Chapter 22

Consideration #3 When Selecting a Dentist

Work with as Few Dentists as Possible

If you ever had a child in sports, you know how annoying it can be to have to take your child constantly back and forth to sports practice.

Sometimes you may even feel that you have no life of your own anymore; your life is nothing more than a constant sacrifice for your child. You don't even remember the last time you did anything pleasurable for yourself.

Now imagine what it would be like if you not only had to take your child to the sports practices, but then take them to an expert in sports psychology who taught them game strategies, then an expert in how to run correctly, another expert in how to get the proper fitting of running shoes/cleats, and yet another for how to recover from those sports practices.

183

Your head would really be spinning, wouldn't it?

It's the same thing with dentistry. Do you really want to go to more than one dentist?

Even if you had to do exactly that, what would you do if the two experts were battling back and forth about each other's treatments, not to mention how much of a gamble you'll have taken on whether you'll like both dentists' staffs?!?

There Are Highly Qualified Type #3 Expert Dentists Who Have Experience in Every Aspect of Dentistry

The answer, of course, is to find a dentist who has attained the necessary education allowing him to do every dental procedure you need in his office.

He has had all the necessary training to do so, and if not, then he has teamed up with another highly qualified dentist who can do what he has not mastered. Because they are working together in one office, they are operating as a team. You feel confident that your teeth are getting exactly what they need.

Choosing a dentist who has to refer you to many other doctors for treatment is almost never the best solution.

Your Biggest Non-Recoverable Asset Is Always Your Time

Jim Rohn, a business sage and public speaker, said, "You can always get more money but not more time." When we apply this to what's potentially happening with your dental visits, you find that being referred to multiple offices "steals" from you that which cannot be replaced: Time!

We all are allotted only so much of it on God's earth, so why let any dentist or other professional waste even a minute?!

For that very reason, our office here in Southwest Florida offers 99% of the dental services that you'll ever need right here in our office.

Full-Service Dentistry Is Available

As a full-service dental practice, Dr. Holtan can help you with all the routine services you would expect, along with the ones that you don't commonly see in most dental offices.

Among the routine services offered are examinations, cleanings, check-ups, fillings, advanced x-rays and computerized dental diagnostics, crowns, bridges, removable partial dentures, and cosmetic dentures.

Among the not commonly seen services are:

* *Dental Implant Therapy*

To replace missing teeth and rebuild smiles, we perform all aspects of the treatment, surgery, and restoration.

Virtually Unbreakable Implant Teeth

New types of porcelain and tooth design make the implant teeth nearly impervious to breaking and chipping.

* *Cosmetic Dentistry Services*

Smile makeover based on computer-assisted Smile design gives you the look you've always wanted. The additional assistance with the computer gives us even greater insight into the creation of a smile that fits you like a glove.

* *Rapid Power Whitening gives you white, bright teeth in about an hour.*

* *Super strong tooth-colored materials* so teeth don't look gray or dark at the gum line…giving natural-looking teeth

Don't settle for teeth that look gray or dark at the gum line, as this result will age you a minimum of 10 years. Who wants that?

* *Full cosmetic consultations* for challenging, difficult situations – restoring smiling and chewing to how they should be.

When you need this type of dental work, it is truly life-transforming.

* *Advanced Computerized diagnostics* for jaw, joint problems, and physiologically based dental reconstructions.

This is absolutely essential when there are difficult dental situations, especially ones where regular dentistry has failed to make a difference.

* *Advanced 3-Dimensional X-Rays*

These are definitely one of the biggest advancements in recent modern dentistry. The ability to see your teeth in three dimensions is a way of ensuring that nothing is missed. They also allow faster treatment and more predictable treatment again based on the many unknowns that are eliminated by seeing your bone, gum, and tooth structure in all dimensions and without any surgery!

* *Dr. Holtan's complete treatments* have saved many patients from unnecessary appointments and sometimes months of time.

* Customized Cosmetic Dentures

* Digital Oral Cameras

These cameras allow you to see what your dentist sees when he looks into your mouth.

Why Not Have One All-Encompassing Dentist?

Many patients say they really like the fact that they don't get sent all over town for their services.

And who wouldn't?

If you have complex dental problems, we even have free "talking" visits to see if your problem can benefit from a customized option by Dr. Holtan.

Now I feel better and look better than I have in years. Have more confidence in myself. Cannot put into words how much this means to me. You and your staff put me right at ease from the first day that I met you. I had very little pain. In fact, I worked during my healing period. I would recommend to anyone that has trouble with their dentures to have implants done.

–Ada, North Fort Myers, FL

Chapter 23

Consideration #4 When Selecting a Dentist

Find a Dentist Who Makes Office Procedures Easy

– In Fact, Makes Them Painless!

Have you ever gone to a dental office and ended up spending hours trying to correct billing mistakes or dealing with insurance company issues as a result?

Or have you ever been to a dental office where they double booked you and you were sent home, only to return at another time? You had spent a good hour traveling back and forth, and really didn't appreciate the lack of concern about your time that had been wasted.

Your New Dentist Should Take Care of All Your Billing

and Scheduling Needs and Do This Painlessly!

In this crazy, modern information overload age, going to the dentist needs to be easy. We and our team hate confusion and complexity. That's why we have spent hours determining ways to simplify all the details for you regarding billing, insurance, fees, and scheduling.

At the office of Dr. Holtan in Southwest Florida, we recognize the importance of being able to get appointments and having a flexible schedule.

We Often Find That Patients Don't Understand

Their Dental Insurance Policies

No Surprise Here as the Policies Are All Confusing!

We help you understand the fees, billing, and insurance so you can be comfortable financially, too. We work to make fees affordable while helping maximize your insurance coverage.

We can do this because we have "learned the ropes" by dealing with thousands of patients' insurance plans over the years.

The best way to help is to file the forms for you, helping you win in dealing with insurance companies. Dental insurance, while not a pay-all, can be a real help in paying for maintenance dental care. But if you don't understand your insurance plan, you can't access the benefits you are entitled to.

We Guarantee to Maximize Your Dental Insurance

For patients with a mouthful of complex problems, we have a 100% guarantee that your insurance plan's maximum will be used.

We help you to get what should be coming to you.

There's one more thing that we make sure of. Our staff wants your total dental experience to be the same we'd want for ourselves.

And the last thing we want is to have to battle for every last cent on an insurance plan. That's just not fun, and – have you noticed? –

the sooner in the day you start to battle with the insurance companies, the more your day is ruined? Who needs that? Let us take care of your insurance claim needs.

Chapter 24

Consideration #5 When Selecting a Dentist

Make Sure Your Dentist Thinks About Your Teeth for the Rest of Your Life

So far, the considerations to make when choosing a dentist are:

➤ **Consideration #1 – Make sure the initial visit is free.**

Otherwise, you could end up with a bill you never wanted and shouldn't have had to pay. And really, why should anyone pay to see if a dentist is a good match for you? We'll get into more of the reasoning on this shortly.

➤ **Consideration #2 – Make sure your dentist has a proven track record.**

Otherwise, you could end up with archaic methods and procedures that cause more pain than what you should have to endure or procedures that are not long-lasting in their effects.

> **Consideration #3 – Work with as few dentists as possible.**

Otherwise, you could end up in the middle of a battle of wills between dental professionals and feel as if you are tossed back and forth with no continuity. You will also likely find that one staff you get along with and the other one you dread seeing at every visit. Never a good situation when one is considering more complex types of dentistry!

> **Consideration #4 – Find a dentist who makes office business procedures easy – in fact, makes them painless!**

Otherwise, you could end up wasting far too much time dealing with insurance companies and their billing staff, wasting time with double-booked appointments, and tearing your hair out with billing errors and have to prove that you are right.

The next consideration is to only work with a dentist who is thinking about your long-term smile and oral health. If he's only focusing on what's happening now, there is a good chance that down the road risks that you have (we all have different risks for types of problems) will create problems that may have been preventable.

Thus, Consideration #5 is this: Find a dentist who thinks carefully about long-term smile health and long-term oral health.

How to Find a Dentist Who Thinks

About Your Teeth Long-Term or from a "Lifetime Perspective"

Now the big question is: How are you going to scrutinize the dentist to find out the answer to the question: What are you thinking about my teeth?

The answer is that this will come out in your first visit with your potential new dentist.

What Should Happen at Your First Visit?

At the first office visit, there are certain topics that must come up in discussion:

• Your past medical history

• Your dental history

• An actual discussion about your lifetime risk in the following six major dental categories:

✓ Gum risk

➢ Risk for changes in your gums.

✓ Cavity risk

➢ Risk for additional cavities forming on your teeth.

✓ Bone Risk

➢ Risk for changes in the foundation around your teeth that supports them.

✓ Smile-Esthetic Risk

➢ Risk to dental work that is visible to you and others especially in regard to longevity of the dentistry.

✓ Bite

➢ How the teeth fit together for chewing and whether there is risk to dental work prematurely wearing out.

✓ Joint Risk

➢ The tendons, joints, and muscles act as a unit to operate the jaw in all of its positions. Do you have risk for some part of the unit having problems?

At your appointment, it's important to express your concerns and what is important to you about your teeth and your treatment. It's important to explain what your experience has been because this will provide clues about how your dentistry and teeth are likely to hold up as time passes. Bare your soul about these; the more you tell, the more your dentist better understands your needs.

If your dentist does not discuss "lifetime risk" as applied to these major 6 dental categories, or seems confused by what you are asking, or tells you this is not important, please be advised to seek a second opinion.

A Dental Examination Is an Important Part of the Appointment

Once you are past the "meet and greet" stage of the professional relationship, it's important for your new dentist to perform a very thorough dental examination that leaves no stone unturned. Think of it as a physical exam for your teeth, gums, bone, joint, and head and neck muscles, as well as facial appearance. A Type #3 Expert Level Dentist will call this examination a "Complete Dental Physical" examination.

We know from experience that many times hidden, unknown problems exist that you don't know about simply because you don't know they are there!

That's why your dentist will evaluate your teeth, gums, and bite, looking for hidden signs of problems that don't hurt until it's too late.

We'll offer you the kind of dentistry that we would want for our own families. We'll help you get the bright, white smile you've always wanted.

We'll answer your questions and work out the needed appointments to give you the best results as quickly as possible while maintaining quality care.

Now that we know that serious, life-threatening risks to your health can be a result of untreated dental problems, we'll help rid you of a dental infection.

You Have a Right to Know the Best Options

You will receive an individual, customized plan of treatment that serves four functions:

1) Correcting your problems

2) Enhancing your appearance

3) Creating long-term solutions

4) Preventing future problems by giving you maintainable dental health

5) Making sure you understand what happens if you choose to do nothing

In most instances, there will be multiple options including a very best option, a very good option, and an acceptable option. By asking your dentist if he would perform a particular option on himself, family member, or loved one, you can also determine if this is someone who really has your best interests in mind. If the answer is yes, great; it's likely the dentist has your best interests at heart. If the answer is no, then once again it could be time to seek out a second opinion or to try another dental office.

We pride ourselves in only offering options that we'd happily see our closest friends and family members choose or would even happily select for ourselves should we need the same professional services.

Once your treatment (if any) is complete, we'll help you maintain your dental health with periodic visits on a schedule designed for you as an individual and based on your lifetime risks.

Dentistry is a lifetime need. Teeth don't heal themselves. If they did, no one would lose any teeth.

Because of our expertise and experience, we often are called upon to deal with very difficult, challenging dental situations.

Every age has its own special dental problems. As you live longer and work later in your life, your dental needs are unique. We help you regain lost function, eliminate painful conditions, and enjoy a youthful, radiant smile.

It is critical that every tooth and every potential procedure be looked at from a lifetime perspective. The reality is that some treatments many dentists do harm the teeth and make them more prone to loss later on, but not at Dr. Holtan's practice in South Florida.

Every Dentist, Including Us, Is Not Right for Everyone

We also want you to know we aren't right for everyone.

In fact, here's a short list of those who are not a right fit with us:

✓ Anyone who does not want to keep their teeth for a lifetime

✓ Anyone who does not want their teeth to look good and to feel good

✓ Anyone who does not want their finished smile to turn heads and receive compliments

If any of these describe you, then it's probably not a good match. If, however, you want to keep your teeth (or new teeth) for a lifetime, want your teeth to not simply look good but to feel good too, and you want your smile to turn heads and command compliments, then it's likely you would find a good home with us.

Dr. Holtan & Staff,

Thank you for all your kindness during my illness with cancer. Frank was so right when he said you all were the best! So glad to have the work completed. Thanks again.

– Marcia

Chapter 25

Consideration #6 When Selecting a Dentist

Find a Dentist Within a Reasonable Travel Distance

Beware of "Vacation" Dentistry

Sometimes people have the idea that maybe they should consider finding a dentist overseas to do all their dental work. This is called dental tourism or a dental vacation; it involves traveling to a destination outside your state or province to take care of health care needs.

Some of the dental vacations that people take include destinations to dentist offices in:

• Austria

• Hungary

• Slovakia

• Slovenia

- Mexico
- Costa Rica
- Peru
- Republic of Ireland
- Northern Ireland
- Poland
- Turkey
- Ukraine
- Australia
- Thailand
- Other countries in Southeast Asia

Many people consider dental vacations because they combine them with a holiday. They see it as a low-cost type of dental care.

Although this type of vacation may seem to be an ideal way to get your dental work, dental vacations do have some disadvantages that you may not have thought about.

Here's a list of a few of these:

- Typically, you will need more than one trip to the destination.

- According to some sources, one-day implants are not recommended because of a higher failure rate for travelers receiving treatment in those locations.

• If you have a dental procedure that goes wrong, you'll have to take a trip back to your destination quickly – and plane rates may be quite high to book a last-minute flight.

• In one report from the Irish Competition Authority, researchers found that consumers complained of a lack of pricing transparency. In other words, "bait and switch" tactics are common in that a low price is advertised and once you make the trip and are at the destination in person, the price changes! The real reason why you may not get an accurate quote is that you need an oral examination to determine exactly what is needed for your situation.

• There is almost always less (if any!) legal recourse if your dentist is in a foreign country.

• You risk making an appointment with the dentist in another country and then finding out that the dentist may not be able to do all your dental work.

• Lastly, the "dentist" you wind up seeing may not even have a license to practice dentistry and it's likely that the dental "education" many will have undergone will not be up to first-world standards!

Your best bet really is a Type #3 Dentist within an hour or two of where you currently reside.

For patients in the U.S., Canada, and South America, considering the newest advancements in dental implants (All-on-4 or The Sclar "One Day" Technique, which give you teeth on the same day as surgery), *it is okay to travel to and inside North America* to have the complex portion of your treatment performed.

After you have your new teeth, a competent local dentist in your area can then take over with ongoing maintenance and "check-ups." In some instances, a local dentist can do everything required after the One Day procedure. Our team is skilled at coordinating this very thing.

However, do consider all the other factors discussed in this book that are important for your selection of dentists. How qualified is the dentist, compared to your dentist over here? How will you know that you like the dentist abroad compared to how much you like the dentist in your own backyard?

The Bottom Line on Choosing a Dentist

There are six things to consider in choosing your dentist wisely:

1.   Make sure the initial visit is free.

2.   Make sure your dentist has a proven track record.

3.   Work with as few dentists as possible.

4.   Find a dentist who makes business office procedures easy and painless!

5.   Find a dentist who thinks carefully long-term smile health and long-term oral health.

6.   Find a dentist within a reasonable travel distance. Beware of travel dentistry. If you are planning on traveling to see someone for advanced implant procedures (All-on-4 or The Sclar "One Day" Technique), be sure your dentist has a plan for both during treatment and after you are finished and are back in your own town.

When you consider these key points, you will find an excellent dentist no matter where you live!

For Dr. Holtan and his staff,

On Dec. 9th, Dr. Holtan put my implants in. It was the first time in months/years I had eaten without discomfort, no pain either real or expected when I bit down, and no "wobbling" of the lower denture.

Surely, I wish I had known about the implant surgery years ago. It would have saved me many years of discomfort and embarrassment. The staff office workers, nurses and helpers were wonderful, so kind and considerate. The dental technician that told me how to care for my implants was very good and very helpful. By the way, I am 87 years old and hope to enjoy eating from now on!"

– Margaret R., Venice, FL

Chapter 26

Dental Implants – An Investment in Yourself That You Deserve

Dr. **Holtan's** Implant Dentistry is an *investment in your looks, emotional well-being, and physical health*. Where else can you have an investment that pays dividends 24 hours a day, 365 days a year? Where else is your investment <u>with</u> you, part of you, enhancing how others see and treat you?... Enhancing how you feel?

<u>Enriching the quality and number of your relationships</u>... Increasing how long you live?

Dr. **Holtan's** Implant Dentistry is the result of a passionate pursuit...a tangible zeal to help people have teeth that last a lifetime and look their best in the process.

We're sorry if we sound like we're too excited. It's just that *we feel so strongly about what our team and we do.*

Most People Have No Idea of Just How Important Their Teeth Are!

Or worse, some people have lost all their teeth but don't know something can be done about it. So please forgive our fervor. It is simply that we want to help people. **We absolutely love being dentists. We absolutely love and adore performing this level of dentistry to help people who have the most serious needs.**

We want to help people who can appreciate the magnitude and importance of a great smile and healthy teeth. If you are one, we invite you to join us.

This quote from the late, great Dr. Harold Wirth underscores why:

The mouth in its entirety is an important and even wondrous part of our anatomy, our emotions, our life; it is the site of our very being. When an animal loses its teeth, it cannot survive unless it is domesticated; its very existence is terminated; it dies.

In the human, the mouth is the means of speaking, of expressing love, happiness and joy, anger, ill temper, or sorrow. It is the primary sex contact; hence it is of initial import to our regeneration and survival by food and propagation. It deserves the greatest care it can receive at any sacrifice.

−F. Harold Wirth, D.D.S.

So, there is the explanation of our life's passion for implant dentistry. Thank you for taking the time to read this patient guidebook. We trust you will have found it informative and of help with your decision making related to your dental needs!

Now it is up to you to make the next move. If you would like for our entire team to care for you in South Florida, be you a Floridian or traveling from other states or even countries, you may reach us via the following ways:

Naples Phone Number is 239-593-4915.

Or fax your request to 239-593-4914.

www.NoMoreDentures.net

Sincerely,

Matthew J. Holtan, D.D.S.

Made in the USA
Monee, IL
27 May 2020

Dedicated to helping every patient gain clarity and understanding of the life-changing miracles of modern implant dentistry

This guidebook is written for education and is not intended to replace component professional advice related to medical or dental health issues. Readers are advised to schedule a consultation and seek treatment with a licensed physician or dentist.